MW01230757

How I Escaped the *SICKcare* System

7 Habits for
Chronic Health:

A 7-week guidebook for lasting change

By Tam Ara

PLATYPUS
PUBLISHING

7 Habits for Chronic Health: A 7 Week Guidebook for Lasting Change (How I Escaped the SICKcare System)

Copyright © 2023 Tam Ara, Tamara J. Rodriguez

First Edition: August 2023

All rights reserved.

No part of this book may be reproduced, stored or transmitted in any form or by any means, electronic or mechanical, without the written the prior written permission of the copyright owner except for the use of brief quotations used in articles, blogs, or book reviews. To request permission, contact the author at Tam@WorkWithTam.ca. The author has no responsibility for the persistence or accuracy of URLs for external or third-party internet websites referred to in this publication and does not guarantee that any such content on such websites is, or will remain, accurate or appropriate.

ISBN# 9781962243537

First published by: Platypus Publishing 2023

Author photograph by Mike@Fotowerks.ca"

Disclaimer: All information and advice contained in this book are based upon the research and the personal and professional experiences of the author. It is intended for informational purposes only. The resource is not intended as a substitute for consulting with a healthcare professional, nor as a diagnosis, or treatment, any health condition. It does not intend to guarantee cure or prevention of any health condition.
The publisher and author are not responsible for any adverse effects or consequences resulting from the use of any of the techniques discussed in this book. The information is general and intended to better inform readers of their health care.

The author of this book disclaims liability for any loss or damage suffered by any person as a result of the information or content in this book. Consult your healthcare professional before performing any exercise program or making any significant changes to your diet and lifestyle. It is your responsibility to evaluate your own medical and physical condition and to independently determine whether to perform, use or adapt any of the information or content in this book. Any exercise program may result in injury. By voluntarily undertaking any exercise displayed in this book, you assume the risk of any resulting injury. If you are experiencing a health issue, consult your doctor in the first instance.

Dedication

To my parents, who inspired me;
to my boys, who always support me;
to my beta group for their feedback;
and to you, my reader,
thank you!

Acknowledgments

Special thanks to my mentors on this journey, especially *Ronan Diego de Oliveira*, who helped me build these foundations; *Vishen Lakhiani*, who trained me to use the power of the mind; and *Eric Edmeades*, who changed my relationship with food forever.

Table of Contents

CHAPTER 1

SHIFT HAPPENS!

Are you *sick and tired of being sick and tired*? Don't worry, you aren't alone.

For the first time in our history, the number of individuals suffering from illnesses exceeds those who are in good health. Studies estimate that over 95% of the world's population has health problems. Over 300 diseases and conditions, and 2300+ disease-related consequences… Those statistics are staggering.

It was also me!

For over 5 decades, I had several chronic illnesses with mounting symptoms: Every day was hard…I was exhausted, in pain, and going through the motions. "You're just getting old," I was told…

I WASN'T settling for that! Midlife should be a time of confidence, freedom of self-expression, and joy. I was *chronically ill* … and I wanted to be **chronically healthy**!

But I was in constant pain, had recurrent migraines, respiratory weakness, was gaining weight, had prevalent insomnia, and increasing mental confusion. I had an arm's length of symptoms. I even prided myself on being able to function on so little… Imagine that?

I was on 7-9 medications daily, and the medical system couldn't do anything but respond to my symptoms and prescribe more medication. One for the symptom, one for the side effects of the first medication, and two more for the side effects of the second. Oh, and some steroids to boot! Still a problem…? Add another medication to the list.

Then I was in a significant car accident and off work for a year in physiotherapy, RMT therapy, working with a kinesiologist, and having slow progress. When I hit plateaus, I was told that this was as good as it gets. Yet again, I was told to accept that I was just getting old.

1

I was frustrated. I felt like there was something wrong with me. I was constantly told my immune system was weak but not told how to fix it. I was told my flexibility was poor but not told how to improve it, only how to treat it or accommodate it. I felt like it was innately my fault...my destiny. I was exhausted and feeling hopeless.

Compounding things, I was witnessing "one of the world's best medical systems" collapsing. My GP retired with no replacement (as many are lately), leaving me on my own to hunt for a new doctor in a climate where no one is taking new patients. Nowadays, people are dying because ambulances are overworked and understaffed, and they cannot reach their destinations in time. People die in hospital ERs before they are even seen because of overwork and understaffing. The reality is that the medical system is in crisis. They need our help! Our local hospital ER doctors recently put out a warning that if you are finally admitted to the hospital (after a long wait), you will likely also wait another 48-72 hours before an attending doctor can see you. Shouldn't we learn how to avoid needing their care as much as possible?

Enough was enough! I wasn't prepared to settle for increasing symptoms and becoming another burdensome statistic on the system. I wanted to escape that! At ANY age!

And I knew there was a broader lens that I needed to use. *What if we focused more on **health** than on disease?* I wondered.

I finally took *control* of my health. I realized that putting Band-Aids on individual symptoms wasn't solving anything. I needed to use a **holistic approach** and deal with improving my health at the source of the issues. I wasn't looking for "quick fix" temporary solutions; so often, we adopt behaviours to reach a goal, and once there...we return to old patterns, and goals are lost.

I asked myself: *What can I do to improve my immune system and prevent ending up in a hospital needing life-saving measures? What is the lifestyle that would promote health and healing?* I found the answers, and hope returned.

WHAT'S THE PROBLEM?

Ironically, so many of the diseases that are overrunning our hospitals are sourced from chronic inflammation, and many stem from lifestyle influences. We are dying of preventable diseases! And we are overburdening our medical systems. The healthcare system is a *SICKCARE* system focussed on treating disease. I wanted to escape the *need* for their services. I wanted to figure out how to prevent my symptoms and not just treat them. I also wanted to escape dying from cancer like my mother at 70 or a stroke like my father at 51.

I started where most people do (the obvious choices): nutrition & exercise. But I was disturbed by things I was finding:

"Eat well," we are told, but there is no consistent guidance. I discovered some VERY disturbing information about food manufacturing, marketing, lobbyists, and the careless way they demand our money at the expense of our health. Even the "4 food groups" is marketing propaganda designed by food manufacturers. Food labels and FDA regulations are manipulated to promote purchases...not health. It's a mishmash of conflict.

"Exercise," we are told. Sit for 17 hours a day and burn it up in the gym for an hour, and we're good, right? Does that even make sense? What we NEED to do is break up our modern-day sedentary behaviours. We are told to use exercise for weight loss, which is difficult and temporary! The math isn't great there. It's easier to give up that extra piece of toast in the morning than go for a 30-minute run. Then, how we "look" is often the focus versus improved cardiovascular capacity. Just another mishmash of conflict.

Most people who want to make a change in health look at changing either nutrition or exercise, or both, like I did. And it stops there. Historically, we haven't been taught much else. And little, if any, mention of social connectivity, our connection to nature, how to improve sleep quality without taking a pill, the importance of having a purpose in life, and how to manage our mental health. Any mention of using the power of your brain to aid in healing? I wanted more.

I studied science-based strategies for improving health and the immune system. I learned behavioural design steps to create a lifestyle that would support my goals. I worked under some brilliant leaders in the health arena to incorporate a series of habits that addressed all the areas highlighted by the **CDC** (Center for Disease Control) and the **NIA** (National Institute of Aging) that promote living a long and healthy life. I used simple, practical, and incremental steps in these critical areas to *reset and recharge my entire being.* I adopted 7 lifestyle habits for chronic health. It's not a temporary quick fix. It's a lifestyle design that is completely doable by anyone to improve their vitality.

I am now pain-free, migraine free, have a strong immune system, and no more chest infections. The weight *literally* dropped off, and now I sleep much better. I experience greater energy, happiness, efficiency, clarity of mind, a sense of connection, and a purpose in life. Miraculously, I am also on only one remaining medication, and steroids are a thing of the past. At 55, I am in a better state of health and fitness than I was 20 years ago! See? *SHIFT HAPPENS!!!!!*

My transformation was enormous!

Your body is miraculous. It is like a seed. You take the raw materials (the seed), give it what it needs (nutrient-rich soil, water, sunlight), and nature does the rest. We are the same.

We consume the raw material, give the body what it needs to thrive (water, food, fuel, sunlight, exercise), and let nature do the rest!

But today we operate our body like it is a car. We run it all over town at high speeds until something goes wrong. Then, we take it to a mechanic to "fix" it. Again, we go racing around town again and are surprised when we eventually end up back at the shop for repairs.

Our bodies are infinitely more miraculous than cars. Cars can't heal themselves if we give them fuel. Cars can't fight disease and create a whole new car by replacing old cells with new ones. Your body can!

We have extraordinary power to change and get healthier. We just need to know what to do.

WHY IS THIS SO IMPORTANT NOW?

Well, for one thing, you want and deserve to feel your best. *Your health is your wealth*! We often ignore this idea until something completely debilitating comes along; it's not a priority until you lose it. We learn to accept our daily "symptoms".

However, living life feeling crappy all the time is a crappy life. We want a happy life. We want to offer our loved ones our "best" and not just "what is left". But we aren't taught enough about how to promote health.

Our healthcare business model operates when there is something *wrong*. This is useful, but we need an intermediary step. We need to take control to improve our health as much as possible first. Our bodies are meant to thrive far beyond our 50s and 60s. Most people shorten their quality of life because of a few chronic diseases.

Imagine a tree. At the top, where the leaves are, we have *diseases* (asthma, arthritis, autoimmune disease, cancer, dementia, diabetes, heart disease, and obesity). These come from the tree trunk. The trunk is *chronic inflammation* caused by core dysfunctions (oxidative stress, hormonal dysfunctions, neurotransmitter dysfunctions, immune detoxification, digestive dysfunctions, and musculoskeletal dysfunctions). The roots of the tree are the *causes* of chronic inflammation, which is found in our lifestyles: diet, nutrition, exercise, sleep, stress, relationships, spirituality, environment, toxins, infections, physical trauma, beliefs, attitudes, genetics, emotional trauma, and drugs). We need to have healthy roots, in order to strengthen the trunk and produce healthy leaves.

What if we focus more on health than on the disease? What is the **lifestyle** that would support an increasing state of health? How do we help ourselves achieve permanent positive changes in the body and our health?

Bodies are a whole system, and so we need a **holistic** approach. When you change only one or two things, often, this doesn't work out long-term. There are just too many variables. So, you give up and feel that something is wrong with YOU! When all we really need is a holistic approach.

Our job is to give our body what it needs and protect it from harm. Then, to let nature do its thing. Like a tree, you don't build it and glue the leaves on. You plant it, give it what it needs, protect it, and nature does the rest. We transform our body and health by giving it what it needs, protecting it from harm, and nurturing its natural gifts. Focus on what is good and nurturing it, rather than focusing on what is wrong and fixing that. If you give cells what they need, they will heal themselves.

WHY DOES THIS MATTER TO YOU?

Well, if you always do what you've always done, you'll always get what you've always gotten!

We all want and deserve to live a healthy and happy life. We want to feel more comfortable and be without pain, to heal injuries faster, and to be more confident in our physical capabilities. For most people, addressing only diet and exercise is not enough to be chronically healthy. This 7-week holistic journey is a great way to start achieving better health.

HOW DO WE PLAN ALL THIS?

Data/studies from the CDC (Center for Disease Control) assessed 4 human lifestyle aspects:

1. Can you maintain a healthy body weight?
2. Do you exercise regularly?
3. Do you eat fruits and vegetables?
4. Are you a non-smoker?

Saying YES to all 4 shows an 80% chance of living a healthy lifestyle free of the 4 big chronic diseases.

Data/studies from NIA (National Institute of Aging) regarding how long/well are you going to live:

1. Do you sleep 7.5 hours on average per night?
2. Do you exercise for 30 min per day?
3. Do you eat mostly whole foods?
4. Do you have at least 3 friends that care about you and you can reach out to?
5. Do you have a sense of purpose that gives meaning to your life?
6. Are you a non-smoker?
7. Do you have protected sex with people you don't know?

Saying YES to all predicts you will live healthy until 90 years old on average. Each NO decreases your lifespan.

The plan laid out in this book is based around creating a YES response to these questions. We're going back to basics to create the foundations of health and fitness. It is an incremental process, building step by step, to create a lifestyle that promotes health. Our basic needs play a major role in our lives. The body's 8 physical needs will be embedded in the plan: air, water, sleep, quality food, physical movement, sunlight, nonenergy nutrients, and physical touch/community.

WHY 7 HABITS?

Very recently in our evolutionary history, roughly 10K years ago, we moved from hunter-gathers into the agricultural revolution. In the last few hundred years, we've had the industrial revolution. Both created a massive shift in our lifestyles. This caused an abrupt change that our bodies were not designed for. We sit all day and have food delivered to us. We eat non-foods. We ignore our stress levels and our connection with our environment. We even ignore our social needs. All this on chronically poor sleep. We need to go back to basics and give the body what it needs.

7 TYPES OF CHRONIC NEEDS THAT ARE NOT BEING ADDRESSED BY OUR CURRENT MODERN LIFESTYLE:

* *Nutrient richness*: having all the fuel the body needs.

* *Frequent movement*: we were designed to be moving all the time.

* *Sound sleep*: regularity, quantity, quality, restore, and repair functions at night.

* *Inner stillness*: our resistance to stress. Prehistorically, stress alerted us to danger, but it was infrequent. Today our lifestyles are filled with daily stress, and we need to recover from it and be resistant.

* *Deep connections*: social networks. We are designed to thrive in a community.

* *Sync with nature*: the body needs its physical environment; sunlight, gravity, water, etc.

* *Sense of purpose*: having a purpose motivates more self-care.

We will use a holistic approach, adding all 7 habits to our lifestyle. These are simple steps to promoting health and vitality.

In this book we will discover *HOW* to *design behaviours* around frequent movement, nutrient richness, sound sleep, inner stillness, deep connections with others, being in sync with nature, and having a sense of purpose.

And *HOW* this *holistic lifestyle approach* can change your body and mind, your overall health, and your life in the greater sense. This is for *any age at any stage*. If I could restore my health after 50 years and create lasting change, so can you!

WHY LISTEN TO ME?

First, because I'm just like you...sick of being sick, tired of being tired, and frustrated with being frustrated. Just an average Joe with chronic symptoms who made a MAJOR health transformation! I know what it's like to suffer from illness and injury. But now I know so much is within our power to CONTROL. If I could do it and create lasting change, so can YOU!

8

Second, because I do have a few creds in the health arena:

* I was a public school teacher in the inner city for almost 3 decades. In the last few years, I worked as an integration teacher in special education, dealing with severe chronic health conditions in students.

* I have a master's degree in curriculum and instruction specializing in health education and have been teaching Health Ed curriculum for over 20 years.

* I was commissioned by our government's Ministry of Education to write a curriculum that was mandated to be taught from kindergarten to grade 12 in all schools in British Columbia, Canada.

* I have taught health for years, and I know what is being taught in schools and in society. I know what I believe needs to change for us to sustain healthy and thriving populations.

* I am an internationally accredited life coach, and now I am certified as a Health and Wellness coach, working with clients to improve their lifestyle and transform their health. I have worked with countless clients on mindset, stress management, goal achievement, and now on using a holistic approach towards health transformation.

* I have studied under, and been certified to teach by, some of the leading experts in health and fitness, nutrition, and using the power of the mind for accelerated healing.

So, are you ready to reclaim your health? Let's make **SHIFT HAPPEN**!!

We start by talking about rabbits...

CHAPTER 2

DON'T HABIT LIKE A RABBIT:

A Word On **Habits**

Habits are YOU! Whatever your **habits** are, they reflect who you are and what you value. What is important to you? You are here reading this book, so I can assume that becoming the healthiest, happiest version of yourself is the goal. And we all know that "nothing changes...if nothing changes". We are here to change *something* in order to improve our state of wellness. We need to start by being observant.

> *Watch your thoughts; they become words.*
> *Watch your words; they become actions.*
> *Watch your actions; they become habits.*
> *Watch your habits become character.*
> *Watch your character; it becomes your destiny—*
> **Lao Tzu**

This is a book about habits. Having said that, there is a bit of housekeeping that we should start with.

In order to evaluate the effectiveness of any changes you make, you need to know where you are at. What is your starting point, your *baseline*? Otherwise, how will you know how far you've come? *Awareness* is the key. It's one thing to know where you want to be, but if you don't know where you *are*, it sure makes it harder to get there, doesn't it?

When you think of your day, what are some of the habits you already have? What are your habits around food choices, exercise, and sleep? Make a list of these habits. Now, think of the *trigger* for those habits you've identified so far. What leads you to make those choices? What time of day do the habits occur? Finally, think about each habit. Which are helping you, moving you towards your goal? Which are not? Is there anything your body says NO to that you do anyways? (We aren't changing anything yet!! We are just building some awareness before we start)

OK, now that we *have* some awareness of where we're at, do you have your glasses on? Lean in close...**this is important:**

I have found that THE number one thing people do wrong when trying to adopt new habits is that they try to make **too many changes too quickly**. We rush the first steps. There is a sense of urgency that we need to make the changes *yesterday* because we've let things go to the point that we are desperate.

Inevitably, we can't keep up with all the rapid changes, so then we give up on changing our lifestyle. Or we do it for a short-term goal (losing weight for a wedding), adopting rapid changes that get results but aren't sustainable. Then, we end up going back to our old habits afterwards and get right back to where we started...or worse. This is a sign of an *unconscious transformation*.

If you are anything like me, I know you may be tempted to adopt EVERY habit we explore and try to check off ALL the boxes. Scan through all the chapter recommendations and plow ahead at top speed. I will caution you against that. *Too much too fast* is **not sustainable.** You will burn out! We have the rest of our lives to keep building. Remember the tortoise and the hare? *"Slow and steady wins the race."*

We need to decrease the sense of urgency and realize that this is a continuous journey; it is not a sprint, a short-term solution, or a magic pill. Being healthier is the by-product of building a healthier lifestyle. There is no "quick fix", so to speak. There are, however, many things under our control that can produce rapid changes for the better. The body is built to be efficient. We just need to help it along a little.

We will be using a *conscious transformation* model and working on *behavioural design* to make wise choices and make the action steps easy. We will discuss these more as we go.

So, let's slow down our sense of urgency and enjoy the journey. The chapter sequence is specifically designed for transformation, and I encourage you to follow them in order.

Another important factor to keep in mind is that we are NOT aiming for perfection. Life isn't perfect, and we shouldn't expect ourselves to be perfect, either. What we CAN do is commit to ourselves that each day we will do our best. Recognize that "best" may alter from day to day. Some days your best will be better than others. And that's ok. What is not productive is to expect perfection in ourselves and then give up because we didn't do that *one thing* perfectly today. It's the perspective that says, "Oh crap! I ate a bag of cheezies! I blew it. I can't do it. I guess I'll just go eat crap from now on." Instead, we will get back up!

I will share some strategies in a further chapter, things like creating **Safety Net Routines** and **Get Back Up Routines**, that will help you plan for when life takes over. You never have to be perfect in an area before you move on. You just need to do the best you can for yourself because you are WORTH IT!

This process requires patience. Not huge patience, as I noticed things changing for me quite rapidly. But patience, nonetheless. Results don't happen overnight. The cumulative result of your daily actions and your habits requires consistency and some time. Good things are worth waiting for! But if you stick with it, within 7 weeks, I predict you will notice many improvements and changes, some of which you may not even expect.

You'll never change your life until you change something you do daily. The secret of success is found in your daily routine.
John C. Maxwell

Your habits determine your future.
Jack Canfield

Some other things I've learned about habits along the way:

* There is a difference between *identity-based habits* and *outcome-based habits.* Outcome-based is temporary; identity-based creates lasting change.

* The brain needs habits so it can free up energy to work on problem-solving, etc.

* There are cues, cravings, responses, and rewards.

* New habits you want to adopt need to be:

   Obvious (make it visible; put the fruit you want to eat more of in a bowl on the counter);
   Attractive (something you want; choose your favourite fruits, use a pretty plate);
   Easy (take incremental steps; eat one more fruit per day than last week), and
   Satisfying (makes you feel good; enjoy the taste and how you feel afterwards)

* Conversely, habits you want to eliminate need to be:
   Invisible (hide the cookie package in the back of the top cupboards);
   Unattractive (buy cookies for the family that you don't like);
   Difficult (don't keep cookies in the house; go out to get one if you must have one), and
   Unsatisfying (remember how eating too many makes you feel)

* It is also important to try not to break the chain. A habit missed once is an accident. *A habit missed twice is the beginning of a new habit.*

So, HOW DO WE DO ALL THIS?

There are 3 strategies we will use throughout this process:
1.   **The theory of marginal gains** (1% improvements)
2.   Zero Resistance Habits
3.   Habit stacking

1.   THEORY OF MARGINAL GAINS:

I'm sure you've heard of 1% improvements. It is also known as the *Theory of Marginal Gains*. *David Brailsford*, a British cycling coach, brought his team to victory during the 2012 Tour de France by using marginal gains.

Have you read **Atomic Habits** by *James Clear*? He explains the math: If you get 1% better each day for a year, you will end up being 37 times better by the end of the year. Conversely, if you get 1% worse each day for a year, you will decline nearly down to zero. He says, "In the beginning there is basically no difference between making a choice that is 1% better or 1% worse. (In other words, it won't impact you very much today). But as time goes on, these small improvements or declines compound and suddenly you find a very big gap between people who make slightly better decisions on a daily basis and those that don't". (pg18)

If you are working under the mindset that small decisions, small choices, and that little thing you are going to do right now won't have an impact on a larger scale, then *think again*! Let's aim for 1% improvement and watch what happens. BABY STEPS!

Our second tool, one of the fundamental strategies we will use to encourage our habit-forming capabilities throughout our journey, is to develop *Zero Resistance Behaviours/habits*.

2. ZERO RESISTANCE HABITS:

The key to change is taking small steps in the beginning. Find the path of least resistance for your new habit. These are "micro-steps" forward.

For example, let's say you want to create a morning routine. The first step in a zero-resistant habit is the easiest thing possible to do. Every morning when you wake up and put your feet on the ground, you say, "*Let me do great things today*". Can you imagine doing this? It's the shortest morning routine ever. A microstep! But it creates the space for your morning routine, a spot on your schedule. Later it can be expanded.

We focus on incremental steps. If you are wanting to start an intermittent fasting routine of 16 hours, start with a small step. Trying to begin with 16 hours right off the bat is a major challenge. 12 hours is what most people do anyways; try 8 PM to 8 AM. It is likely a step of "zero resistance" for you. IE "I can do that!" Then try 13 hours, then 14, and build your practice step by step until you reach 16 hours comfortably, without resistance.

The point is to make starting the habit as easy as possible and build incrementally towards the goal. "Slow and steady wins the race". Be the tortoise, not the hare!

CREATING A ZERO RESISTANCE HABIT: (the Fogg MAP method)

Stanford professor *BJ Fogg* explains that behaviours / habits are a product of 3 things. As long as we have:
Motivation (your WHY, reasons for doing the behaviour),
Ability (to execute the behaviour), and a
Prompt (that triggers the behaviour), then the behaviour will happen.

Therefore, behaviours are something we can "design" and control. This is *fantastic news*! It is the fundamental pillar of this book. We CAN effect change for improvement through a conscious transformation by intentional design. We can create a "recipe" for any behaviour we want to adopt.

Creating a **"recipe" for behavioural change** includes:

* Choosing the lifestyle improvement you'd like to develop.
* Brainstorming ways to achieve the goal.
* Identifying the highest impact actions on the list.
* Checking in with your body: are you open or resistant towards the behaviour? How can you make the habit easier?
* Choosing the action you are open to and ready to try.
* Finding a prompt. Usually, the best triggers are those that are already in your environment. Use the habits you already have in your day for prompts.
* Adding an immediate celebration. This is *crucial*. It reinforces the behaviour and creates motivation for doing it again. If you don't signal to your brain that the event is important and worth repeating, it will not respond as easily. The "celebration" primes the emotional habits releasing dopamine which fuels our motivation to repeat the behaviours. Long-term rewards don't strengthen your habits. It needs to be immediate.

* Rehearsing **X 7**. Seriously, DO IT! Act it out physically. This is the make-it-or-break-it part. Here is where we are *programming* the brain.

This has been a monumentally helpful strategy for me in creating my own transformation, and I invite you to put it into your toolbox as well.

Add to this: another of the most helpful things I learned from *James Clear* was the practice of "**Habit Stacking**".

3.   HABIT STACKING

The premise here is that it is easier to add a new habit when it is stacked on top of a current habit. There are 3 steps to habit stacking.

* Set an "*implementation intention*": what you want to do.
* *Stack your habit:* add a new habit after an existing habit.
* Then add *temptation bundling*: Make it attractive and irresistible (Premack's Principle: behaviour is more attractive if we get to do our favourite things right after).

I highly encourage you to try this system when building your new habits over the next few weeks.

And now...are you ready? Let's go slowly, make 1% improvements each day, build one zero resistance habit each week, and stack our habits for success.

We will start with awareness...the key to change.

YOUR TURN: Homework Time

1.   Habit awareness

Sometimes we're stuck in patterns or habits that aren't supporting our transformation or goals. Let's start by identifying the habits that are in place:

When you scan through your day, what are some of the daily habits that aren't helping you? (*e.g., food choices, exercise, sleep habits, social isolation*). Don't try to change anything yet! First, we are only trying to understand the things you do and/or things you don't do that are taking you in the opposite direction and aren't helping you reach your goals.

If you have trouble identifying habits, start with the following:
* How do you start the day?
* What are your habits around meals right now?
* What are your habits around movement throughout the day?
* What daily routines show up?
* How do you end the day?
* Which habits are supporting you and which are not?
* When do these habits happen in the day?
* What leads you to choose the behaviours that you've found so far? Can you identify the prompt for those habits? What is the conversation that happens in your mind that leads you to choose those behaviours? i.e., What triggers the choice?

Habit	Trigger	Time of day it happens

What does your body say NO to, but you do it anyways?

Please note: you're not changing anything yet...just being mindful as you are going through it.

Now that you know where you are, remember 1% improvements and make a commitment to yourself to go slowly. Perfection is NOT the goal.

2. Create Zero Resistance Habits

* Pick one goal to start.
* Choose the habit to be added.
* Brainstorm 10 different behaviours, microsteps you can see yourself doing, that could achieve that goal.
* Identify the 3-5 highest impact behaviours from the list.
* Check-in with your body (check your reactions). Choose an action you are open to trying.
* Write the recipe. IE: Add your *external prompts*. *Stack your habits* (instructions below). Add an immediate *celebration* (reinforces the behaviour, creates motivation)
* Rehearse the whole process 7 times...act it out!

Bonus #1: Want to start early? Add this first new zero resistance habit:

The shortest morning routine EVER!

* Get out of bed and put your feet on the floor. Say, *"Let me do great things today!"*
* Add a victory pose, a phrase...like something you say to celebrate your team's scoring. Maybe it's "YES!" or "Oh YEAH", a high 5. I use one from a hilarious old video game called WORMS: I hold up V with my hand and say "Victory" in a funny worm character voice. Sometimes I do it discretely if others are around...LOL.

Easy, right? Can you see yourself doing this? It's a baby step that is DOABLE. But it sets you up with the *real estate of time* to start building other habits.

And finally, for all our new habits moving forward, we will use the *Habit Stacking* method for lasting change.

3. Stack your habits (recipe)

i. Set an *"implementation intention"*:
I will (behaviour) at (time) in (location)
Set your cues (time, location, make it visible)

ii. Stack your habit:
After I (current habit), I will (new habit)

iii. Then add *temptation bundling*:
After I (new habit), I will (tempting behaviour)
Make it attractive and irresistible.

So, for example, it looks like this:

Implementation intention (1)
+ habit stacking (2)
+ temptation bundling (3)
=

1. I will do a **workout** at **6 AM** in the **home gym**
2. After I make my **smoothie**, I will do my **workout**
3. After I do my **workout,** I will drink my **smoothie**

Finally, remind yourself of what you're trying to accomplish by visualizing often and over time. The more you visualise it, the more it becomes part of your self-identity, and the easier it becomes to continue the habit effortlessly. Meal times are often used as a prompt for this practice in many, many cultures around the world. It is a powerful time.

Bonus #2: add this second bonus habit: **MVP**

Try a *Meal Prayer* or **Meal Visualization Practice** (MVP), whatever you choose to call it.

For example, during one meal of the day:

*Take 6 deep breathes to activate the parasympathetic nervous system
* Visualize yourself achieving your goal. Experience the feelings you will have at that moment when you achieve it (we will revisit and expand on this practice in later chapters).
* Express gratitude for being in this place.
* Visualize the action steps it will take to get there.
* Create a little mantra/prayer that resonates with you (e.g., "Let it be so", "amen", etc.)

WHAT'S NEXT?

All this seems doable right? There *is* a little bit more to revamping our habits. We often don't change our habits unless we address our *self-identity*. There's a lot that goes into this part.

If you find along the journey that you are struggling with resistance and commitment, this will likely be the obstacle. You may need support here to unpack it. It is a personal and individual journey and, as such, is not covered in the scope of this book. Reach inside and explore, discuss with a trusted support person in your life, or feel free to reach out to me at Tam@WorkWithTam.ca, as I have many tools to help and am eager to assist you in this area.

Are you ready? I'm excited for you!

Let's set our intentions:

* I commit to giving my body what it needs, protecting it from harm, and nurturing its innate gifts throughout this journey.
* I will go slowly, making 1% improvements, listening to my body to choose my goals, using zero resistance habits, and using intentional behavioural design towards improvements.
* I will observe my baseline, monitor my progress, and celebrate all my successes.
* I am in control, and I deserve this.

Ready for week one? Buckle up... Let's go!

CHAPTER 3

ABOUT LAST NIGHT

Week 1: Sound Sleep

If we are starting from the beginning to build a strong health foundation today, we need to talk about last night. How did you sleep? If you're anything like I used to be, maybe it wasn't all that great.

I had always been a notoriously BAD sleeper. "Sound sleep" was not in my vocabulary. I was that gal at work functioning on 3 or 4 hours per night and plastering a big smile on my face saying, "It's as good as it gets, nuttin' I can do." I was up all night gasping for breath as a lifelong asthmatic or tossing and turning from arthritic pain all night. I spent HOURS lying awake in bed waiting to fall asleep…and HOURS up in the middle of the night trying to "get tired" enough to go back to sleep. Neither staying in bed nor getting up was helping. But I was so used to it that I discounted my own behaviours that were contributing to the problem.

I was just a BAD sleeper. Period. My whole life. I don't remember *ever* sleeping through the night until well into my adulthood. I learned at the surprising age of 17 that most people "sleep all through the night without waking up"….WHAAAAAAT? I really thought my condition was normal, and all the medical professionals later in my life gave up trying to help me improve it. I was even sent twice to an overnight sleep study with no result.

"We don't know why," they said. "Here, take these pills for sleep." So, I gave up too.

However, I was also a religious coffee drinker. I NEEDED it! Because I was a bad sleeper, remember? Ridiculous. They used to call me "Two-fisted Tam", as *everywhere* I went, I'd have 2 coffee cups with me…yeah, seriously. When I was a teacher, my son entered kindergarten at *my school*. The kindergarten assignment (draw your route to school and back home) produced an uproar of laughter in the staff room one day.

"What's so funny?" I asked as I walked in on the laughter.

"One of the kids drew Home to Starbucks to School, and School to Starbucks to Home."

"Oh, hilarious," I said. *"Which child?"*

"YOURS!" was the answer. They only found it so funny because it was so true. I later scaled down to Tim Hortons coffee due to cheaper cost. I should've taken out shares in these companies. But "Oh, no... it doesn't affect my sleep".

(Side note: Although caffeine wasn't always changing the amount of sleep I was getting, it definitely changed the archetype of my sleep. Less REM sleep left me feeling groggy when I awoke and all day... unless I had more coffee. And the cycle got worse...)

My case was extreme. I was waking over 35 times a night and in bed for many more hours than I was sleeping. But I resisted the idea of "regular sleep schedules". I would succumb to sleeping in, napping, and going to bed early, all to compensate for the previous night's poor sleep. I *lived* for these accommodations. It's part of the pop culture of working people, right? Live to stay up late on weekends and sleep in or nap. Turns out it was the WORST thing I could've done.

Well, things got even more dire for me during menopause, and I knew I really needed to get a handle on this beast. People started talking around me about sleep, and I discovered that I wasn't alone. Research shows that now about 1 in 7 adults experiences insomnia, and for women, stats are about 1 in 4. I had already invested a lot of time researching and learning, and I solved a lot of my issues. Not great, but better. Then menopause hit, and well...

WHAT'S THE PROBLEM?

The main problem with chronically bad sleep is that your body's natural daytime and nighttime processes, your circadian rhythm, get interrupted. Nighttime is for *"rest and digest"* functions of the body. This is when all growth, healing, and repair take place; sleep is the environment in which it happens. Brain cells communicate, and toxins are removed from the brain. These are critical processes for performance. If this is interrupted, you are shortchanging your body's ability to function. Things start to break down. Additionally, if you lack sleep, you tend to gain more fat and lose muscle. Your circadian rhythm needs to be balanced to reduce chronic inflammation.

There is a whole lot of science out there about what sleep IS, the sleep stages and cycles, and learning your chronotype for sleep. If you are interested, I invite you to explore. But for now, the main thing we need to know is that:

The main goal of sleep is to *balance your circadian rhythm and reduce chronic inflammation in the body, to rest, digest, grow, and repair.*

So, HOW DO WE DO THIS?

First, we evaluate the baseline: where are you at right now? On average, how much sleep do you get each night? How long are you in bed? Try a sleep tracker journal.

Then, look at the big picture. What are your goals? Be specific and realistic. Visualize achieving the goal.

We can start by improving the *quality* of sleep. Let's face it, getting 10 hours of interrupted poor-quality sleep leaves you feeling worse than 7 hours of good-quality sleep. You may find that after working on improving the *quality* of your sleep, you actually need less sleep than you thought in order to feel refreshed and ready to go each day. I used to think I needed 10 hours to feel good. Now, I regularly get about 7, and I feel better than I ever have.

After that, we can work on *quantity* if needed.

To improve the *quality* of our sleep, we start by adjusting the following:
1.   External environment
2.   Internal environment

3. Sleep schedule

Let's start with the easy stuff: *Optimizing the sleep environment and minimizing sleep disruptors.*

1) EXTERNAL environment:

* ***Be cool!*** Our bedroom needs to be at a cool temperature. In order to sleep, our body needs to be able to lower its temperature. If your circadian rhythm is balanced, your body temperature will decrease automatically around your bedtime. If not, cool your room down. Optimum temperatures are between 16-20 degrees Celsius. (60-67 degrees Fahrenheit).

* ***Be dark***! Our brain registers *light* as "daytime", including blue light from devices. We need to perceive darkness to release melatonin, the sleepy hormone. Try *blackout curtains* or a *blindfold* to eliminate light entering your eye receptors.

Extend your "blue light free time". Stop using any devices 1-2 hours before bed. Start with a small step, like 30 minutes, and extend your time up to 2 hours. Some people have success with *blue light blocker glasses* when working on devices later in the evening.

Are you feeling some resistance here? Find out what emotional attachments you have to giving up blue light; look for substitute behaviours that meet that need. For example: What emotion are you looking to feel? How else can that goal be fulfilled? You watch TV for entertainment? Play a card game. You email others or scroll social media to connect? Call someone or visit with your living companions.

Create prompts (after I brush my teeth, I will play a game with my kids) and *eliminate triggers* (after 9 PM I will put my devices away in my office for the night).

Keep evening lighting at a height below your eye level; use table lamps instead of overhead lights. This lower-level light triggers your brain to register "evening".

* ***Be quiet!*** Noise-free and distraction-free. Try earplugs. Some people find white noise helpful.

24

* _Be in bed ONLY for sleep or sex_! No reading, emailing, scrolling, watching TV, phone calls! Any time you do any other activity in bed, you train your brain to expect the same in the future. It conditions your brain to think of "bedtime" as the time to read or connect or work. How can you possibly expect to sleep soundly at your "work desk"? Separate your other activities OUT of your bedroom and start to condition your brain to expect sleep when you hit the pillow at night.

* _DON'T spend time awake in bed_! Try tracking your time spent awake and asleep in bed. I came across a sleep journal (I'll reference it at the end of the chapter) that has the most comprehensive tracking chart I've seen. Some use fitness watches to track sleep cycles. Tracking really helped me identify how long I was lying in bed restless and contributing to my problem. I discovered that I was in bed for 10 hours but only asleep for about 3 - 4. That information made me finally prioritize my sleep habits and make a change. Awareness is everything, right?

* _Cold shower in the morning_ also helps to balance our circadian rhythm. Start with a few seconds and build up to 2 minutes per day.

2) **INTERNAL environment**: the harder stuff!

* _Reserve nighttime for Rest and Digest functions_. Stop eating 3 hours before bedtime. Digestion takes an enormous amount of energy and effort from your body. It raises your body temperature. It also produces insulin, thus reducing the production of melatonin, our sleep hormone. It isn't possible to grow and repair while we are digesting. Give your system a break from processing calories and the space to receive the benefits of the nutrients you've consumed. Especially take a break from high-carbohydrate foods late in the evening, which can contribute to the number of times you are waking up at night.

* _Avoid stimulants_. Yes, that means coffee. I see you cringing...I did too. I was EXTREMELY resistant to giving up coffee. You may have guessed. However, although it may not keep you up all night, it definitely changes the archetype of your sleep, preventing REM. Alcohol, too...sorry guys.

* *Create a wind-down routine.* Trigger your body to expect sleep. Unwind with mindful practices, inspirational reading, a quick yoga or stretch session. And stay OUT of bed until it's time to sleep. You will train your brain to associate bed with relaxation (sleep or sex only).

* *Clear and calm your mind before sleep*. Try an "Unload Journal" to write down all the thoughts running through your mind. Use paper and pen, not your phone or computer, so you don't activate blue light exposure before bed. Write down all those endless thoughts, tomorrow's plans, reminders, and worries BEFORE you get into bed. Let them go. They can wait until tomorrow.

Now, the hardest stuff!! But it's the most important. We can look at getting enough *quantity* of sleep. This also improves the quality of your sleep and all your body processes. This is done by:

3) *REGULATING your sleep PATTERN*.

And that means...get ready! (maybe you should sit down). You need to...**Go to bed and get up at the same time EVERY DAY!**

YES, even on weekends! Seems a little counterintuitive, doesn't it? Weekends are for sleeping in and naps and "catching up".

I *know* this is tough! But changing your sleep schedule to accommodate a poor night's sleep (sleeping in, going to bed early, napping) contributes to the *next* poor night's sleep! It completely dysregulates your circadian rhythm. There is so much to this that I could write another book on sleep alone. But you will have to trust me here. Take it from a chronically horrible sleeper for the past 5 decades...this WORKS!!!!

I no longer have to be so particular with my sleep environment or the other adjustments because my circadian rhythm is balanced perfectly. Please give it a chance. Really! If you adopt nothing else from this chapter, DO THIS!

STEPS TO REGULATING YOUR SLEEP:

1. Observe the earliest "commitment" you have during the week. Is it getting the kids to school every day by 8:00? Getting to work by 9:00? The weekly morning Zoom meeting at 6:30?
2. How long is your morning routine? If it's 2 hours to shower, eat, and get everything ready to start your day... set your alarm for 2 hours before your earliest weekly commitment.
3. Then set an alarm for 8 hours and 15 minutes prior to that. *This is your new bedtime*. For **EVERY DAY of the week.** THIS is imperative. Keeping a regular schedule is what makes the biggest impact on your energy, your digestion, and everything else.
4. Do your evening routine without devices.
5. Activate your parasympathetic nervous system (rest and digest) by using controlled breathing strategies. At night we need to access the parasympathetic nervous system. The main tool to accomplish this is to use our *breath*. Breath is the connection between our unconscious mind and our conscious mind (our automatic functions and those we can control.)

Exercise: 4 – 7 – 8 Breathing
* Get ready
* Breathe in for 4 seconds
* Hold for 7 seconds
* Breathe out for 8 seconds
* Repeat steps 2-4 eight times

6. DO NOT adjust your sleep schedule to accommodate a poor night's sleep, or you will continue to dysregulate your circadian rhythm. Going to bed and getting up at the same time each and every day is the very best thing you can do to balance this rhythm and help your nighttime healing processes function effectively.
7. Here is where you *can* adjust. If you wake up before your alarm feeling refreshed, perhaps go to bed 15 minutes later and try that schedule. If you wake up feeling groggy, perhaps go to bed 15 minutes earlier.

8. *Adjust* until you find what *your body* needs. On average, we need about 8 hours, but some people need 7, and some need 9. We are all different. This process will take time and your patience, but it is *the biggest impact action you can take to improve your sleep quality and quality.* Trust the process here.

Some side notes here for your further study if it interests you:

Menopause: During this time, we are stepping into a different body because hormones are changing, and things are different. We might need different strategies. For example, our natural calming functions are less effective because our progesterone level is lower; therefore, try to reduce consuming stimulants (caffeine, alcohol, etc.) Be more diligent with your sleep habits. Try a cooling pad on the bed. Many people recommend eating more organic soybeans to slow hot flashing. During menopause, estrogen production (which has a role in reducing body temperature and stabilising moods) slows down, making us hot and irritable. Tough conditions for a restful sleep. Add night sweats, hot flashes, bladder issues, restless legs, anxiety, and disordered sleep to the mix and well, we can see that additional attention needs to be placed on regulating sleep during menopause.

I ended up working with a menopause/sleep expert. If you find, after implementing as many of these strategies as you can over some time, that you need more support, please do seek it. It makes such a difference to my overall being to be well-rested. I can't believe I functioned for so long on so little. I want this for you too!

YOUR TURN: Homework Time

Start by evaluating where you are at with your sleep. What is the big picture? What are your goals? Set realistic goals and action steps for improvement. Be specific; track progress; and visualize achieving the goal.

Look at the areas of Sound Sleep skills; where is your main opportunity (managing your external environment, internal environment, or regulating your sleep schedule)? Choose **ONE** thing you will do this week to strengthen your inner stillness toolbox. If you have a level one practice already, try level two or three.

Action steps/habit building

Level One:

* Evaluate where you're at (how much time in bed, how much sleep / awake time).

* Set detailed, realistic goals and visualize them as having already been achieved.

* Create a wind-down evening routine.

Level Two:

* Eliminate stimulants.

* Address your internal environment.

* Address your external environment.

Level Three:

* Reduce blue light exposure at night.

* Balance your circadian rhythm. Regulate your schedule and adjust until you find your "fit".

* Explore further study if you need more support.

WHAT'S NEXT?

All this sounds simple, but it takes practice. Consistency is the key here. I really didn't think things could change for me, but they did! I dropped the caffeine, stopped eating 3 hours before bed, adopted a wind-down routine, practiced mindfulness and journaled, managed my external environment, and, most importantly, I regulated my sleep schedule. Then, my sleep quality went up, and my quantity needs actually went down.

Address the area first that you feel will yield you the best results. Start with baby steps. Remember, changing too much too quickly is **NOT sustainable.** You can always add more when you are able to maintain and ready to scale up in this category. When you adopt level one practices, move on to levels two and three as you are ready. Remember, quality comes first and then quantity (which often falls into place when the quality improves).

It wasn't a quick fix for me. I worked with *Debs Wallbank,* a menopause specialist and sleep guru, and learned so much. She made me *knowledgeable,* and I can now help YOU learn faster than I did. But she is an *expert*. She has an amazing sleep journal (that I mentioned earlier), a free 3-day Sleep Masterclass, a Sleep Zone Membership, and individual coaching and consulting. She is amazingly fun to work with as well. Check her out if you need more than this; she is someone who's been there and who specializes in helping menopausal women, and others sleep like a baby. Give her a shout: Debs@menodebs.co.uk, and www.menodebs.co.uk

Now that we've slept well and are up and ready for the day... let's get moving!

CHAPTER 4

YOU'VE GOT TO MOVE IT! MOVE IT!

Week 2: **Frequent Movement**

You've heard it: Sitting is the new smoking! But the solution isn't as complicated or time-consuming as we've been led to believe. We don't need to pump iron for hours at the gym each day and run a marathon every week to be fit. I spend no more than 20 minutes on a "workout" session 5-6 days per week, and one session is literally 4 minutes long. You have time for this!!!

We are designed to move. Only recently has our species been afforded the luxury of settlement and constant food production. We were designed to walk all day to find food, shelter, etc. Now, we don't have to. Modern society has us sitting for 10, 12, or 16 hours a day. We sit at the table to eat. We sit in our cars or on transit buses for an hour or more to get to work. We sit at our desks for 8 or 9 hours a day. Return home voyage of more sitting. When we get home, we are tired. We sit some more.

All this sitting has grave impacts. A study (*John D. Akins et al., Journal of Applied Physiology, 2019*) shows people who sit all day and then do one hour of exercise in the gym *gain almost no metabolic benefit* from the exercise. The Mayo Clinic found those who sit for 8 hours or more a day with no physical activity have a risk of dying similar to those posed by obesity and smoking (*Mayoclinic.org/sitting*). A Centre for Disease Control and Prevention study (*"Association between sitting time and cardiometabolic risk factors after adjustment for cardiorespiratory fitness, Cooper Centre Longitudinal Study 2010-2013".*) published in 2016 of cardiometabolic risks discovered a relationship between prolonged *sedentary* time and increased risk for chronic conditions and premature mortality for both men and women.

* As soon as you sit, all the energy going towards your legs isn't needed, which means less blood sugar is being processed by the body.

* When sitting, the body also decreases its release of the protein "lipoprotein lipase" by 90% (an enzyme crucial in breaking down fat into energy.)

* Every hour after you sit, your metabolism rate (rate of energy burn) drops by 90%. Calorie expenditure reduces to 1 calorie per minute.

* 2 hours after sitting, your "good cholesterol" HGL drops by 20%.

* Studies show that after sitting an entire day, there is *no metabolic benefit* gained from 1 hour of exercise afterwards.

* Detriment to the metabolism compounds the longer you sit.

Even our brain needs us to move. Luckily the best movement for us is the easiest. The best thing we can do for brain function is... Ready?

WALK!

Puzzles and number games are all great for keeping the brain active as we age, but the best way to keep the brain active and performing is to walk. After we walk, we experience a 20% increased learning capability. Want to learn something new? Go for a walk first. It produces BDNF (brain-derived neurotrophic factor), which acts like a brain fertilizer. Neat, eh? Other movement activities like stretching are great, but they don't give the brain the benefits of increased heart rate.

Many other studies show strong correlations between improved mood (feeling better and happier) as well as maintaining a healthy BMI when we are active walkers.

The point here is that what we need to focus on is **breaking our sedentary patterns** during the day. There can be a lot of conflicting information out there about how much exercise and what kind of exercise and for how long to exercise, and for how often...just confusing. But in reality, it isn't. You just need to MOVE! And move often using the basic functions your body needs to perform in life. We need to build routines that give the body what it needs to flourish. We need the state of energy flow stimulated by movement. But where to start?

First, what are your beliefs about fitness? Do you think things like... *it's not for me, it's only to look good, it's a superficial goal, I can't be fit, it is the only thing that matters, fitness is a creative expression*? What are *your* beliefs? Some of these are signs of what we call "unconscious fitness". We want to make a *conscious* transformation.

Examples of Unconscious Fitness Attitudes:

* I only do it because I want to look good at that wedding. (*Outcome-based goals yield temporary results*)
* If I can't do it, my life has no meaning. (*Obsessive thoughts negate listening to the body*)
* It makes my life harder; I don't like it, but I have to. (*Obligation-based thoughts lead to a negative association and decreased motivation*)
* I just need to get it done. (*Checklist focus negates the enjoyment*)
* I need to punish my body for training to work. (*Punishing thoughts negate body signals and can lead to injury*)

Examples of Conscious Fitness Attitudes:

* I develop fitness to lead a fully expressed life (e.g., to play with my kids, go surfing, play tennis, go on vacation, challenge myself with a marathon).
* Exercise is an expression in the face of challenge. Fitness helps reduce my stress. It is part of being "unshakable".
* It helps to make my life easier (to have more endurance or power for climbing stairs, lifting groceries, better mobility, less risk of injury, and progression training raises the bar for what challenge means and makes things even easier).
* Physical activity gives me an opportunity to engage with my body, to be "within", and to connect and listen.
* I do it to celebrate what my body can do, to appreciate and expand my capabilities.

We will be *conscious* on this journey, listen to our bodies, and increase our capacity to perform physical functions to make life easier. Our body is our vehicle to experience life. It is a partnership, and we need to be respectful. Give your body what it needs, and it will give you what you want.

THE BASICS

There are 5 areas of fitness we need to develop in a comprehensive, *holistic approach*:

- Muscular *strength*: the ability to lift heavy objects.
- Muscular *endurance*: the ability to keep up strength activity for a period of time.
- Cardiovascular *endurance*: the ability of the heart/lungs to efficiently deliver oxygen to organs, increasing energy level.
- *Mobility*: the ability to move your body around your joints.
- *Body Composition*: percentage of fat vs. lean body mass (water + muscle + bone)

We work on these areas by adopting **BASELINE BEHAVIOURS:**

* Move often.

* **Challenge muscles** with something heavy for a sustained time (around 20 minutes).

* **Stretch muscles** in their range of motion.

* **Provide protein** for recovery (the raw material to build muscle).

* **Give adequate rest** for growth (the environment for growth is sleep).

HOW DO WE DO ALL THIS?

There is a lot to putting this together, but it's worth it. You CAN do it. How do I know? Because I did it. And I'm just an average Joe like you.

After a significant car accident, which left me in physiotherapy, RMT therapy, and working with a kinesiologist for 13 months, my progress had stalled and plateaued. I was told I was just getting old, and this was as good as it gets. It's what triggered me to start this journey myself.

I listened to my body and worked on progressive baby steps to build a solid fitness foundation. My body is stronger than it's been in decades. The key is really listening to your body signals and going slowly to prevent injury. So, what to do?

#1 We can WALK!

How much to walk? Well, you've likely heard of the 10K step rule. Funny, as wonderful as that number is ... It's a bit arbitrary. It was a number set by the first fitness monitor manufacturers because their device could count up to 10,000. Yeah…really. It's a great number, but realistically, somewhere between 7000 and 10,000 is a good goal.

Aim for above 7000 steps. Below 7000 steps per day has been shown to expose you to a greater risk of chronic disease. Additionally, at least 3000 of those steps should be done at a brisk pace to *raise your heart rate* and improve cardiovascular endurance. A brisk 30-minute walk first thing in the morning is an easy way to accomplish this. If you want to track your numbers, use the step tracker on your phone if you have nothing else.

How often to walk? If you aren't walking, you're probably sitting. *Frequency is important. Getting 7000 steps is a good walking goal.* A 10-minute brisk walk is about 1000 steps. If you did 30 minutes in the morning and 20 minutes after lunch and dinner, you'd be at 7000 already. Add to that your daily moving about, and you'll be getting all the benefits!

What *else* should we do? *Try to break your sedentary behaviour every hour!*

#2 Break sedentary patterns

Every hour or two do a **MICROWORKOUT**. This is one of my favourite strategies: 1-2 minutes every hour to break sedentary patterns. We need 3 basic functions from our body. We need to be able
1. *to push*
2. *to pull*
3. *and to squat*.

Find a version of each of these 3 exercises that you can perform accurately. There are a TON of YouTube videos that are great for finding these. Test the versions first. Find one within your current capability. Then, do each version until you hit fatigue (when you cannot do one more repetition accurately). Record the maximum reps you can do.

Take your *maximum number of reps* per exercise (push, pull, squat) and do *50% in 1-2 minutes*.

For example, if your maximum reps for push-ups is 20, do 10, and for squats, if it is 30, do 15. Repeat reps cycling through the various exercises until you reach 2 minutes. Push, then pull, then squat, then push again, pull...and repeat.

Add any other cardio exercises you like. 20 Jumping jacks, 5 burpees, etc., for variety. Just keep moving for 2 minutes. You are getting the blood flowing, raising your heart rate, and working on muscle strength, all while breaking the sedentary pattern, all in 2 minutes!

Come on now, *everyone* has 2 minutes!

Strength = 50% muscle + 50% skill. This practice increases the motor function/skill for these exercises, which helps to increase your maximum capacity. In other words, you are not trying to increase performance; it is not a progression session. The main purpose is to break the sedentary pattern and to raise the heart rate. You can use this multiple times a day to break sedentary patterns and raise your metabolism.

Exercise (squats, push-ups, pull-ups, etc.)	Maximum reps in a row	50% of maximum

#3 Increase our *Baseline Fitness Behaviours*: *SHOW UP Sessions*

Do you have some way of exercising the 5 areas during the week? If so, FANTASTIC!

If not, we can start here: Add a *place in your schedule for your daily* "**Show Up Sessions**" of 20 minutes. Remember to "listen" to the signals/sensations your body sends you. Consult your healthcare professional if you have injuries before starting or changing a fitness routine. We will focus on *baseline strength, baseline endurance, and baseline mobility* routines in the course of a week.

Of course, I do other movement, or "workout", activities besides strength, endurance, and mobility training (hiking, biking, kayaking, paddleboarding, dancing, etc.), but these are for enjoyment and are not "training" for *progression*. I *train* to get stronger so I can do these other physical activities that I enjoy so much.

Do some research on some fitness routines that cover *strength training, cardio, and mobility*.

I found a 6-day program that covers 2 days of **strength** training, 2 days of **endurance** interval training, 1 day of **mobility** training, and 1 for cardio. Each session ranges from 10 – 20 minutes for a full workout. My cardio training is literally 4 minutes!! Yes...4!! Check out Tabata endurance training for a super-efficient routine!

A) BASELINE STRENGTH

The muscle advantage! Working on building strength is the MOST important factor in your routine as it has a cascade effect on all other areas. If you do nothing else, DO THIS!

Developing more muscle mass:

* *Controls your blood sugar* (blood sugar causes the most inflammation; this also regulates our metabolic health). The more muscle you have, the faster your body can take the sugar out of your blood and reduce the chances of *inflammation and insulin resistance.*

* *Prevents/reverses muscle loss* (as the body is exposed to more stress, it responds by building and maintaining muscle).

* *Prevents sarcopenia*. This is a progressive and generalized loss of skeletal muscle mass and strength. Risk factors include age, gender, and activity level. We need to exercise enough to show our muscles that they are needed. If you aren't using your muscles, they conserve energy, lose mass, and then we have even less energy and strength to use them.

* *Builds bone density*. Keeping bones strong prevents serious injury during falls. The average loss is 1% of our bone mass per year after age 40. If bone density is fragile, falls are very dangerous. About 60% of people who break a hip are not able to regain independence. But you *can* regain muscle mass that has been lost.

* *Supports your joints*. Stronger bones have less tension on the joints. Strength training, especially for those with arthritis, can relieve symptoms by using a slow progression-based training program.

* *Burns more fat*. Burning fat helps with body composition. Muscle is like a furnace, and it burns more calories if it has more mass.

How our body burns energy:

* **Basal Metabolic rate**: 70% of our energy burned is based on our metabolic rate.
* **Non-exercise activity thermogenesis:** 15% of our energy is burned on the amount of activity we do throughout the day.
* **Thermal effect of food:** 10% of energy is burned on digesting the food you eat.
* **Exercise activity thermogenesis**: ONLY 5% of energy burnt during the day comes from exercise efforts.

In other words, if you are using exercise to burn energy and lose weight, only a *5% result* comes from that. It's much more efficient to raise our BMR by increasing our muscle mass. Boosting the 70% efficiency level instead of the 5% is more productive for weight loss goals. Therefore, strength training is one of the most effective ways we can get our body to burn more fat.

Strength training also:

* Improves posture and emotional support. Think about the postures you use when you are in a low state. Hunched shoulders, looking down. And how else do you *feel* when you are in that posture? Physical manifestations can evoke emotions. Think about being on the computer or phone all day in hunched postures. It is easier to feel sad if you are already hunched over. Unfortunately, it also builds the musculature of "hunch". We need to build a skeletal musculature of "upright".

* Improves all biomarkers of aging. Strength training improves your **biological age** (how much your body has aged vs. your chronological age, the amount of time since your birth). Have you ever noticed how one person can look like they are 40 years old when they are 50, while others look like they're 60 years old when they are 50?

It is important to remember the *3 Main Functions* we need to perform in life: **PUSH, PULL, SQUAT.** We will start our training for strength, endurance, and mobility here.

Look for some instructional exercise videos for strength (push, pull, and squat) and ***find a version*** that you can do at least 8 repetitions. *If you can easily do 12, then you need a harder version of that exercise. If you can't do 8, find an easier version*. Push-ups can be done inclined on a wall, on stairs, or on a counter. Find one that is challenging but doable.

Once you have chosen your versions for each of the 3 areas that you can do 8 – 12 reps in a row, do the exercise to find the MAXIMUM number of reps you can do (when your muscles fatigue and you can't do anymore.) Record your maximum reps for each.

Next, schedule 3 Show Up Sessions for the week: **2** Progression sessions (where you look to increase performance slowly step by step each week) and **1** Study session (where you search for other versions of exercise, or perfect your technique, etc.).

	PUSH UP	PULL UP	SQUAT
Maximum			
Time / Day for Show-Up Sessions			
Type: Progression or Study			

Training for *Progression:*
* Find your form of the exercise.
* Find your maximum repetition number.
* Do each set stopping 2 reps away from failure. If your max is 20, do 18.
Each set of repetitions includes:
     1st set: do squat, push up, pull up, stopping 2 reps away from complete failure.

     2nd set: repeat sets *4x until your maximum reps for each exercise is compl*ete. For example, if your max reps in a row for squats is 10, your total goal is 40. Complete sets until you reach 40. The example below shows 5 sets until max is reached:
1 = 10
2 = 10
3 = 8
4 = 8
5 = 4

     Next time during your weekly strength training, increase your goal by one rep per exercise. When you easily reach 3 x 12 reps in a row, try a more challenging exercise. Find your maximum and repeat the process.

The 3 Main Exercise forms to explore (have a search on YouTube):

PUSH Up Exercises
- Level 1 Wall
- Level 2 Incline
- Level 3 Full
- Level 4 Side to side

PULL Exercises
- Level 0 Australian Pull-up (gymnastic rings attached to pull-up bar)
- Level 1 Inverted Row Pull-Up (on the ground with a broomstick and 2 chairs)
- Level 2 Assisted Pull Up
- Level 3 Negative Pull Up
- Level 4 Full Pull Up

SQUAT Exercises

- Level 1: Partial range of motion – touch the edge of a chair and stand up
- Level 2: Full range of motion – go all the way to the floor
- Level 3: Lunge
- Level 4: Split squat – lunge with one leg on a chair
- Level 5: Archer squat – lunge to the side
- Level 6: Pistol Squat – 1-legged squat

B) BASELINE ENDURANCE:

The strongest benefit of endurance training is brain health. It stimulates the growth of new neurons. Brain oxygenation promotes clearer thinking, more creativity, and learning capacity boosts by 20%. Increased heart rate seems to play a role. Incorporated into your daily routine, developing endurance promotes continued brain health and prevents early deterioration.

Cardiovascular disease and respiratory disease are among the top killers on the planet today. Endurance practices increase our heart and lung health. It also regulates blood pressure.

Walking briskly can achieve this goal. Try *interval walking*: brisk walk for 2 minutes, regular walk for 1 minute, brisk walk for 2, etc. You just need to get your heart rate elevated to experience the benefits of cardiovascular exercise.

What else do you enjoy? Swimming, hiking, biking? My endurance activities are some of the most fun in my weekly rotation. When I do them for progression, I track my performance and work towards step-by-step goals. Schedule *1 Show-Up Session* each week for *endurance training.*

Endurance exercise:
One option:
* 20 minutes of sustained effort
* Raise heart rate to a specific level

* Keep elevated for 20 minutes at a moderate level (when it's a bit hard to have a conversation)

Your targeted heart rate: Be safe while you are doing *it!*
Heartrate goal equation
(220 – your age – your resting heart rate) x 0.6 + your resting heart rate)
EG (220-55-65) x0.6 + 65 = 125bpm

Interval training:
If you can't manage sustained effort, try interval training alternating between high and low paced activity. For example:
* 1 min run, 1 min walk for 20 minutes.
* 1 min fast walk, 1 min normal walk for 20 minutes
* 1 min uphill, 1 min downhill for 20 min.
* 1 min jumping jacks, 20 sec rest (add burpees or side shuffles, etc.)
The goal is to reach 1 min of exertion and 20 seconds of rest. Go for progression.

C). BASELINE MOBILITY

What mobility exercises do you need? First, identify what is the limited range of motion, if any, that your body has. Where are your limitations? These may be uncovered during your *Show Up sessions.* Notice what feels difficult or stiff:

*Is the squat exercise difficult?
* Is your back hunched?
* Is it hard to lift your arms over your head?
* What is difficult or impossible to move?
* What is stiff? What are the daily limitations of the movement?
* Where are you "immobile"?
* What shows up for YOU?

If you have injuries, it's best to work with a physiotherapist on this.

Then, dedicate a **Study Session** during the week to *explore all kinds of new exercises*. Perhaps a 30-day yoga challenge. Find where there is resistance. YouTube has Yoga Challenge series, qi gong, stretching, etc. Find an exercise that matches your limitation and add it to your schedule. Maybe add a Sun Salutation to your morning routine.

Build a routine of stretches and exercises that increase that area of mobility you want to address.

Your weekly schedule might look like this:

Show Up Session #	Day of the week	Focus	Reflections
1	Monday	Strength: Progression	
2	Tuesday	Mobility (recovery; try things out)	
3	Wednesday	Strength: Study	
4	Thursday	Endurance	
5	Friday	Mobility (recovery; your routine)	
6	Saturday	Strength: Progression	
7	Sunday	Rest	

* Try adding a mobility movement component to your **AM routine**. I use a 15-minute Qi Gong routine I found on YouTube that I love! It gives me energy, gets my body fluids moving, encourages flexibility, and gets me ready to start the day.

YOUR TURN: Homework Time

Look at the areas of frequent movement; where is your main opportunity (increased walking, microworkouts, baseline fitness routine)? Choose **ONE** thing you will do this week to strengthen your frequent movement toolbox.

* Note: If you are looking to make body composition changes, you MUST take your biomarkers first to track your progress and stay motivated. Take ALL of these. It is MUCH more motivating to see **all** the changes, not just traditional measuring that tracks only the chest, waist, and hips.

Weight	Shoulders	Waist	Calf
BMI	Chest	Hips	Ankle
Body fat %	Arms	Thighs	
Neck	Midsection/bellybutton	Inner knee	

If you have a level one practice already, try level two or three.

Action steps/habit building:

Level One:

WALKING 101

* Analyze where you're at: spend a few days keeping track. Do you have a step counter? Phones often do. If not, an average "guestimate" is about 100 steps per minute. A 10-minute walk = 1000 steps.

* If you are below 7000 per day, how can you incrementally increase that number? Create Zero Resistance habits; try adding 5 minutes to your walk at a time. Create the space for "the walk" in your schedule. Try 10 minutes after each meal. That's 3000 already. Walk during phone calls. I often do my best "thinking" while I walk, and I take memo notes on my phone.

* I do a brisk 30 minutes in the morning before breakfast / 20 minutes after lunch / 20 minutes after dinner, and that's my 7000 already. That's my baseline: then I add walking the dog with my boys or seeing a friend for a forest walk whenever I can. Plus, all the incidental walking during the day, parking further away, taking the stairs, all that other stuff that you know.

* Most importantly, start building incrementally. If you're not in the habit of daily walking, don't try to add a 30-minute and two 20-minute walks right off the bat. Start with 10 min and add 5 minutes every few days. Going *too far too fast* is **NOT SUSTAINABLE!**

Level Two:

* MICROWORKOUTS: a 1-2 minute Micro-Workout: (short, far from your max, but enough to raise heart rate). Do **50%** of your maximum reps in the span of 1-2 minutes (e.g., Max squats 16? Max push-ups 24? Do 8 squats, then 12 push-ups.) **Add** various exercises that raise your heart rate on repeat until you reach **2 minutes.** Use multiple times a day to break sedentary patterns. Cover push, pull, squat, and any extras you choose.

* **Expand your Morning Routine** (Are you still doing the shortest morning routine ever? "Let me do great things today!") Now is the time to add a bit of gentle movement to set you up for the day. Find your favourite video. I like a 15-minute Qi Gong routine that covers all the bases.

Level Three:

BASELINE FITNESS ROUTINE

* Set your schedule for Show-Up Sessions:
- Strength training/progression training
- Endurance training
- Mobility training

Choose your activities. Track and monitor your progress.

* Continue to increase your goal in progression sessions by 1 repetition per exercise. Once you reach 3x 12 reps...try a more challenging version.

* Do PROGRESSION sessions x 2 per week and 1x STUDY session, which is the most important for improvement. Research new videos for flexibility.

WHAT'S NEXT?

All this may seem overwhelming at first, especially if you are just beginning. It was for me. I wanted it ALL...all at once. But that is NOT sustainable. This is DOABLE and sustainable IF you pace yourself. If I could do it after a major car accident, so can you.

Start where you are at and go SLOWLY in this area in particular. Consult professionals where you need to. Remember, it is not a race. Address the areas first that you feel will yield you the best results. Start with baby steps. Changing too much too quickly is dangerous here. Your body needs time to adjust to changes. Be respectful of the relationship. You can always add more when you can maintain and are ready to scale up. Move through the levels as you are ready.

So, now that we're up and moving … **let's get outside!**

If you still are wanting more, here are some areas to consider exploring:

Mindset:
* Discover the body: what feels easy? Any pain or discomfort? Limited range of motion?
* Observe the mind: "I'm weak"; "This will take forever"; "Going nowhere"; "Feels great"; "Looking forward to ME time". What beliefs are reflected in your mind chatter?

Scaling UP:
* What are your fitness goals?
Movement = physical activity
Exercise = the movement you do to improve something
Training = all exercises done with a specific goal in mind

Training VS Workout
A *workout* is a lifestyle choice that puts our bodies in motion. The benefits are variety, overall health, and it's good for you.
Training is designed to achieve a specific goal. The benefits are from a structured program with targeted results. And it's GREAT for you!

* Exploration of more *functional fitness exercises* (push, pull, squat, walk, carry, lunge, deadlift, resist, twist)
* There are complex distinctions for *training levels* (i.e. 2x effort does not always = 2x benefit)

* For efficiency, try *compound exercises* (working multiple muscle groups in one exercise)

Other considerations…

Women with a cycle: first 2 weeks are more intense (try doing 60-70% of your training in the first 2 weeks, 20 % in the third week, and 10% in the last week.)

Differences during menopause: hormonal environment changes significantly. Estrogen (bone density, muscle protein synthesis, cognition, insulin, joints, temperature, fat distribution) and Progesterone (mood regulation, sleep, balance, and grounding) sink to an all-time low and stay there for the rest of their lives. Training should focus on strength training (to address weight gain, muscle loss, osteoporosis, and insulin resistance.)

Explore on Google: self-assessment for pelvic floor questionnaire (also app 'Squeezy").

CHAPTER 5

LET'S MESS WITH MOTHER NATURE
Week 3: **Sync with Nature**

As I write this chapter today, I sit in my backyard oasis enjoying 29 degree Celsius, *clear sky* weather. And THAT is a blessing. Now, this makes more sense if you know that I live in Vancouver, Canada. A rainforest climate...and I may be biased, but I would venture to say it's the most beautiful place on earth. It rains a LOT, but that is what makes the landscape so brilliant. Now I have traveled to a mere 2 dozen countries, but I cannot find a place that has it *all* like my home. You can go skiing in the morning, hike a mountain trail in the afternoon, and cool off with a dip in the lake or the ocean in the evening.

I've never taken it for granted. Even though I live in one of the biggest developing cities in my region, it is a "City of Parks". I can walk to one of our *most* beautiful parks, where we have forest trails, riverfront views, fields of wildflowers, and snow-capped mountains in the background, and I can walk there within 10 minutes. I walk every day. In my neighbourhood, I enjoy the cherry blossoms, the neighbours' gardens, and the little stream near the park. On a longer venture, I go to other parks, beaches, forests, river frontages in neighbouring areas.

During COVID restrictions on cross-community travel, it was tough. We could walk our pets but only within our immediate neighbourhood. You could visit a park, keeping your distance, wearing masks, and only within a certain radius from your residence. It was hard being kept away from some of my favourite haunts, but I learned to appreciate my little neighbourhood more. As with everything, there is beauty to be found if you look.

But I am concerned. Having worked in schools for the past 3 decades, I have seen changes. Children increasingly don't play outside like I did when I was growing up. There are several reasons for that. Safety concerns, neighbourhood dangers, longer working hours for parents, and also devise-based engagement or entertainment...many things.

I believe I grew up as part of the last "free-range child" generation. It was the 70s, and children played outside until sundown. Neighbourhoods were safe, and we were allowed to roam free until the mother serenade began, "Johnny....Diiinnnneeeerrrrrr!" We got dirt under our fingernails...hell, we ate mudpies. We breathed in the soil. If we didn't get dirty, well, then we didn't have fun. It bred a certain immunity to germs and disease.

Environments are "super clean" now. Kids don't build the same kind of immunity that we did by being exposed to dirt and to animals. Before COVID, we tried to veer away from the *hand sanitizer movement* in schools because they had been shown to have an adverse effect on children's developing endocrine (and other) systems. Now, during and post-COVID, we can't seem to get enough of hand sanitizers. I propose that we have become "too clean" in our obsession to be disease free. We need to go back to basics and reconnect with the environment we were born to thrive in: the natural environment.

We were designed to "be in" our environment; we need sunlight, oxygen, and gravity. There is so much to gain from being attuned and aligned with nature. Seems easy...but are you doing it? Besides the pure enjoyment of it... there are so many benefits to building habits of reconnection with the earth.

I know, I know. You don't have time. Well, let me tell you, at the point in my life where I had NO time for anything and was burning out...the forest brought me back so I could function again. My mother was in the hospital with weeks to live, and I had been there 20 hours each day for 2 months, back and forth driving home 30 minutes each way only to shower and maybe eat. I didn't want to do anything that would take away my last hours with her.

But I was suffering. My boys insisted they take me to the forest when they saw how I was crashing. 30 minutes sitting at the creek literally gave me the strength to carry on those last really hard days. It cannot be overstated the power of nature. So, let's remember that NOTHING is as important as you and your health. If you don't have that,

you can't be there for the ones you love. Let's go play outside!!!
EVERYDAY!

HOW CAN WE DO THIS?

1. Get outside and experience the benefits of nature.
2. Collect "places" that rejuvenate you.
3. Get "outside" yourself and help protect the earth.

#1 JUST GET OUTSIDE!

Here are 10 ways you may not be aware of that we benefit from being in nature from *NatureConnectionGuide.com*:

a) **Phytoncides**: Airborne particles are released by *coniferous trees* as a defense against insects, disease, and temperature changes. When we breathe these compounds into our lungs, our NK (Natural Killer) cells and anticancer protein levels increase and remain higher for days. This boosts our immune and can help fight off many diseases. So...breathe deeply next time you're around these magnificent trees.

b) **Bacteria:** Soil contains so many beneficial bacteria, particularly Mycobacterium vaccae, which studies show can lower our stress and anxiety, boost our immune defenses and elevate our mood. Repot your plants, weed your garden, reach down and smell your neighbour's soil bed...and see how you feel.

c) **Feeling in AWE:** Appreciation and gratitude for the beauty that surrounds us cannot be over-emphasised. Being in awe of the power of a waterfall, the serenity of an ocean tide, the majesty of mountains, the caves and forests...it DOES something to us. A research paper exploring the "awe factor" by *Jonathon Haidt* and *Dacher Kelter* in the Journal of Positive Psychology *(2018)* called *The Development of the Awe Experience Scale (AWE-S): A multifactorial measure for a complex emotion,* found these events are one of the most powerful ways we experience personal change and growth. They found we are more generous, ethical, and deeply connected to others as we recognize the interconnectedness in our world. We see ourselves as part of something greater. Go find your AWE spot...make a collection!

d) **Negative Ions:** Negative ions evaporate into the air from moving water (waterfalls, rivers, waves on the ocean, water in forests). The plants also release these ions, which attach to and remove harmful particles like dust, molds, bacteria, and allergens. These ions in the air help improve our cognitive functions, productivity, and psychological health, as well as decrease stress/anxiety/depression symptoms. More reasons to breathe deeply and let nature do its thing for you.

e) **Fractals:** These shape patterns are found everywhere in nature; *even we* are made up of fractals! Our eyes are designed to understand fractals, and seeing them produces a relaxed state, even reducing our stress levels by up to 60%. Physicist *Richard Taylor* from the University of Oregon has written many articles about these benefits. Check him out. Then Google fractal images for examples, but they are literally everywhere: clouds, shells, leaves, pinecones, snowflakes, mountains, flowers, coastlines...

f) **Earthing:** Or grounding (I can't even believe there's a name for this... We used to call it walking... LOL). Walking *barefoot* synchronizes the electrical energy in our bodies with the negatively charged free electrons that come from the earth's surface. We are spending less and less time walking barefoot, so I'd hazard a guess that we all need a little reconnecting. There is talk in the scientific world about the importance of this connection with our sleep, our gastrointestinal symptoms, our pain levels, the amount of inflammation in our bodies, and our feelings of stress. Sounds like a good time to kick off those shoes and walk in the sand, on the grass, in the dirt...let it sink in. Literally!

g) **Sunshine:** Depending on where you are on the planet, the amount of natural light can fluctuate. Many people even suffer from Seasonal Affective Disorder. Sunlight exposure is biologically woven into our sense of well-being. Serotonin, our feel-good hormone (which affects sleep, digestion, appetite, memory, social functions, sexual desire and function), is boosted by the sun. Our skin absorbs Vitamin D to help our bone health, cardiovascular function, muscle function, respiratory function, fight infections, and protect us from cancer. If you get your Vitamin D between the hours of 8:00 am and 12:00 pm, you get the added benefit of balancing your circadian rhythm, boosting your metabolism, and burning more fat. I go every morning before breakfast. Sunny, cloudy...doesn't matter. You still get the benefits either way. Even sitting on your patio for 10 minutes on a cloudy day will do it.

h) **Sound:** The sounds of nature work to keep our bodies calm and out of the *Fight or Flight* response state. Brain functions improve as the sounds physically change our mind and body systems. The "quiet" of nature is also beneficial, giving our brain time for inner stillness. Listen to the birds singing, the river flowing, the waves crashing, the wind blowing, and the insects chirping.

i) **Smell:** Smell activates memories (smelling the soil always reminds me of great times gardening with my grandma) and is commonly used for healing. Essential oils such as lavender, peppermint, and sage decrease anxiety and insomnia and activate the parasympathetic nervous system.

j) **Fungi:** Not a subject to be taken lightly, and IMHO, requires some guidance by "professionals". Psilocybin mushrooms have started to become more widely talked about as a treatment for various ailments. I have no experience in this area, and if you choose to explore, I urge you to do your research and find reputable sources and practitioners to guide you.

#2 COLLECT PLACES THAT REJUVENATE YOU!

Make a list of places you feel benefit from. I love the sound of the water, the smell of the forest, the eel of the grass on my feet. What fills you up? List some options:

* If I have 15 minutes, I will go to...
* If I have 30 minutes, I will go to...
* If I have a few hours, I will go to...

Have some options ready to accommodate different time frames of availability for yourself.

Finally, how else can we be in sync with nature?

#3 GO "OUTSIDE YOURSELF" AND PROTECT THE EARTH!

* **Conserve water**: There are so many options if you look. Low flush toilets, low water washing machines, water-saving shower heads, etc. Some options are cheaper than other. Do some research.

* **Conserve energy**: Consider household reductions, lower your carbon footprint, get energy-efficient appliances and lights, and air dry your clothes.

* **Reduce your meat consumption**: There is huge evidence as to the detriments to the planet around the meat industry.

* **Eat locally**: Cut fossil fuel costs of food transportation and grow your own food.

* **Eliminate:** Get rid of disposables and single-use items. Plan ahead. Use cloth bags, glass containers, and water bottles. Keep a kit in your vehicle or bag so you're always prepared.

* **Resell, reuse, recycle:** Electronics is in the news right now. So much waste is being produced, and nowhere to put it. Just for the latest iPhone? Repurpose what you can, sell what you can, take to a recycling depot what you can, and donate what you can.

YOUR TURN: Homework Time

Look at the 3 areas of Sync with Nature skills; where is your main opportunity (getting out in nature, collecting favourite locations, or protecting the earth)? Choose ONE thing you will do this week to strengthen your Sync with Nature toolbox. If you have a level one practice already, try level two or three.

Action steps/habit building

Level One:

* Walk in your neighbourhood every day.

* Smell the trees, the flowers, and the soil.

* Repot plants or weed your garden.

* Plan a visit to a nature spot that appeals to you this week.

* Conserve water.

* Shop locally.

Level Two:

* Find 3 local nature spots that make your soul happy: Be it riverside, ocean beach, forest trail, mountaintop viewpoint hike, neighbourhood playground, flower gardens, or waterfalls.

* Create your list: when I have 20 minutes, I go to…; when I have 60 minutes, I go to…

* Plant a garden and grow some food.

* Eat less meat.

Level Three:

* Conserve energy.

* Ditch your single-use items and plastics. Replace with cloth bags, glass containers, and glass water bottles.

* Recycle, repurpose, resell, and donate.

* Swap out for energy-efficient household items and appliances.

WHAT'S NEXT?

As I've said before, it seems simple, right? Just go outside. But are you *doing it? Every day?* Address the area first that you feel will yield you the best results. Start with baby steps. Remember, changing too much too quickly is NOT sustainable. You can always add more when you are able to maintain and ready to scale up in this category. When you adopt level one practices, move on to level two and three as you are ready.

So, we've improved our sleep, gotten ourselves up and moving, and gotten in sync with nature... Now, it's **time to eat!**

CHAPTER 6

HOW RICH ARE YOU?

Week 4: **Nutrient Richness**

Oh my, this is a BIG one! Are you ready? I feel like I could just burst over this one... It's hard to know where to start. Take this in small doses this week!

So, let's start with...the D word.

"Diet" has come to be known as that thing we do for a short period of time, some alteration we make to achieve a goal, usually weight loss. Some magic concoction, a mix of strategies, and foods to create a temporary solution to a problem. We "go on a diet".

In fact, our DIET is: a way of life. It is ALL the things we eat. Every living thing on the planet has a specific *diet* that they have evolved the ability to process and have developed dependencies on. Evolution is a slow process. It can take hundreds of thousands of years to evolve different food processing capabilities or different nutritional requirements. Our bodies were designed to eat a full range of nutrients. The more closely we adhere to our evolved diet, the healthier we will be and the less disease we will experience.

But is what we're eating now our evolved diet? During the Agricultural and Industrial Revolutions, we discovered we could mass produce food, and we could make more money from food if we made it tastier. We started to explore the refinement and taste of food. For instance, if we remove some of the fibre in potatoes, people can eat a little bit more. If we remove the nutrients out of seeds, we can make oils. If we refine and process and take out nutrients and give added sugar (which gives fireworks to the brain) we can sell even more stuff. Food-preserving additives mean longer shelf life but more toxins. We created foods that our bodies weren't ready to process and absorb.

We created mass manufacturing capabilities, and food manufacturing was convenient. But we learned to make overprocessed foods, with flavours and additives for "better taste". We created *new foods* of convenience for the busy modern working family. However, much of this "food" is not recognised by the body as food; there are no nutrients it can use to grow and repair. Think of Cheezies, for instance...one of my favourite childhood "foods". How many other "non-foods" can you think of? Much of what we eat now causes physical symptoms:

* Lethargy and fatigue
* Brain fog and lack of focus
* Mood swings
* Gas and bloating
* Constipation and diarrhea
* Joint and muscle pain
* Headaches
* Runny nose and sinus congestion
* Rashes and eczema
* Heart palpitations
* Nausea and vomiting
* PMS and cramping
And the list goes on...

I discovered that my respiratory congestion and wheezing were perpetuated by dairy foods. My arthritic pain and skin rashes are amplified by grains. My headaches are promoted by sugar consumption.

So, why do we eat these foods that cause so much harm? One reason is that we are unaware of which foods are causing which symptoms. We look to treat the symptoms instead of identifying and eliminating the causes. We treat the disease instead of looking to promote health (prevent symptoms). It's not your fault; it's what we've been taught because it's how our healthcare system works. We need to build **awareness** as to what certain foods are doing to our body and awareness of the *types of hunger* we are feeding. We often eat because of reasons not at all related to true hunger.

And yet another reason we eat tasty "non-functional foods" is that we have been taught to "treat" ourselves. Had a bad day? Treat yourself. Had a great day? Treat yourself. Been really "good"? Treat yourself. Been really "bad"? Treat yourself. You need consoling, treat yourself. Doesn't matter what the reason is: *You deserve a treat!* Sound familiar? It's in all the marketing. Your friends and family probably even say it. But think for a minute: You definitely *are* treating yourself. But are you treating yourself well, or are you treating yourself poorly? Hmmm.... YEAH!

If you want the *best* health (because you really do deserve it), then you absolutely deserve to *treat yourself well*. And that means giving your body what it needs and protecting it from harm.

"But everything in moderation," you say? This argument is usually made to justify some non-functional food. And, well, moderation is great, sure, if you want mediocrity. But, as Eric Edmeades points out, a moderate diet results in moderate health. This is why 2 of the biggest killers in the Western world, cancer and heart disease, are often described as lifestyle diseases due to our poor health choices. Still, this is *fantastic* news. Why? Because *this* is something we can control. We need to be aware, and to refrain from making decisions in the moment without considering the cumulative damage that is being caused by your short-term tasty treat. Nothing tastes as good as longevity feels. I don't want moderate health; I want excellent health! What about you?

So, to build awareness, what should we be aware of and pay attention to? BIG question!! Let's start with:

BUILDING AWARENESS

TYPES of Hunger:

* *Thirst*: We often mistake thirst for hunger because, ancestrally, our foods had more water content. Our "thirst" was a signal to eat more (water-rich) food.

* *Nutritional Hunger*: The true hunger signals from our body that we need for nutrients.

* *Low Blood Sugar*: When we haven't eaten for a while.

* *Variety*: We are meant to eat a variety of foods to get all the nutrients we need. We are programmed to need variety. If we eat the same things all the time, we can feel "hungry" even after eating.

* *Empty Stomach*: Some people don't experience this often. An empty stomach isn't necessarily needing more. It just feels empty, and we perceive it as a void to be filled. We live in a "snack culture", and we eat all day long.

* *Emotional:* It's been estimated that at least 80% of our food choices are based on nostalgia. Foods remind us of times, people, and places. When we want to fill an emotional need, we have been taught to fill it with food. Commercials are based on this: they show a warm, fuzzy emotional event and immediately show their product, so you learn to link the emotional state (having a laugh with a family member = love and belonging) with consuming their product. Can a product really make you feel closer to Auntie Joan?

We can help ourselves here by listening to our internal dialogue around food. What are your thoughts as you have a "craving"? What leads you to your choice? How do you feel after making that choice? Often, the *decision* to act gives us more pleasure than the act itself. This awareness helps us recognize our "sales technique". What things does your mind tell you to justify poor choices? Becoming aware of these thoughts makes them less effective for you moving forward.

Now, how do you feel after the first bite? The second? Halfway through? After eating? 4 Hours later? The next day? This can help us identify WHY we are choosing what we do and HOW that choice *actually* makes us feel physically.

Ok, so ironically, I should mention that...food that makes you "feel good" in the short term often makes you feel bad in the long term. But food that doesn't make you feel bad in the long term doesn't necessarily make you "feel good" in the short term. However, there IS hope. Your taste buds will change, and you will soon LOVE all the wonderful foods we will talk about just as much as you loved those Hawkins Cheezies that remind you of road trips with your parents.

A sea of (mis)information:

Our economy is built on an outdated model. We have a trillion-dollar food industry based on selling convenience foods and junk foods. Foods that aren't food at all. There are government subsidies to bring down the cost of the ingredients in those foods. Why aren't they funding fruit and vegetable production, seed and nuts, legumes, etc.??? If we subsidize anything, shouldn't it be what the body actually needs?

There is more manipulation in the food industry than there ever was in the tobacco industry, and yet we all know now that smoking is bad for us. The tobacco industry worked to convince us to take up an *extra* habit, not one we needed for survival. They used manipulative marketing, which we know is bad. They continue to sell a product that causes harm to consumers. However, the food industry uses all the same tactics to manipulate us into buying and consuming junk. And somehow, that's OK...

Here's where it's really bad...The food industry exploits our *basic need* (hunger, we all must eat) and tempts us with dysfunctional, super tasty treats. High fat, high sugar, devoid of any nutrients, kinds of foods. They add "flavours" to compensate for taste and add all the stuff our brain goes nuts for. The combination of sugar and fat sets off fireworks in our brains. We LOVE it! But...at what cost? If you're interested in more, I invite you to watch "The G-word" on Netflix regarding the food manufacturing industry. Seriously! Watch. Quite simply, the food manufacturing process and the resulting "food" created that is void of nutrients is BAD for us. But we're getting smarter. We know the damage these ingredients cost us, so we have learned to read labels.

But they're on to us. Your eyes aren't getting worse; those labels ARE getting smaller. They don't want savvy consumers reading ingredient lists. Did you know there is an acceptable margin of error in labeling the calorie content of products? Yup, up to 20%! Now, I'm no scientist, but that seems like a rather large margin of error. They even rename items to fool us. Did you know there are at least 65 different names for sugar? Manufacturers don't want to list "sugar" because they know we are now looking for it.

Unfortunately, sugar is what makes you LOVE that product and want to buy more. It's addictive.

And it has HUGE side effects. Now, 50% or more of North Americans are prediabetic or diabetic. When I was growing up, there was Type1 Diabetes and Adult-Onset Diabetes (now known as Type 2, which is also called a lifestyle disease.) We don't say Adult Onset anymore because, astonishingly enough, more and more children are now being diagnosed with this disease. I noticed the increasing trend in the schools over 3 decades. The foods we are eating are causing weight gain, among other things. Our populations are becoming "obese" on average. If any of this is news to you, then what they're doing is working.

Above and beyond all the food manufacturing and marketing dangers, we are fed more lies. Pop culture would basically say...eat what you want, and if you gain weight, then exercise is the solution. This was propagated by the sugar and soft drink industries, who funded a research study to prove that fat consumption was the problem, not sugar, in rising obesity rates. Message being... sugar good, fat bad. Their commercials back in the day even showed a woman in workout gear drinking a pop and then going for a run. The fitness industry loved this. People flocked to buy gym memberships, which were ineffective for weight loss, so people kept going and faded off, but more bought in.

The funny thing is that 80-90% of our body composition is based on the foods we eat. The way our body burns fat is 70% through our BMR (basal metabolic rate). Maintaining a healthy BMI (body mass index) increases our BMR and is also important for blood sugar control, insulin resistance, and eliminating belly fat, the most dangerous kind. As we've discussed, only 5% of our results in weight loss efforts come from exercise. Exercise has other obvious benefits (cardiovascular health, muscle and bone strength, mobility, etc.) But for weight loss, it is not an effective solution. In fact, it leaves people feeling bad about themselves because they "can't do it". If we are trying to be efficient, then we should put more effort into the 70% by raising our BMR. And here's where food comes in.

The amount of sugar we put into our bodies is what determines our ability to control our blood sugar. Too much for too long produces insulin resistance, requiring more insulin to regulate the blood. This causes inflammation and weight gain, which lowers our BMR, encouraging more weight gain. Researchers estimate about 70% (or more) of all manufactured food products contain sugar.

But the food industry doesn't want you to know all this and stop buying their products. All they want is your money, and they're taking it at the cost of your health. Manipulating your emotions and falsifying information, and deflecting attention...all at the expense of your health.

You vote with your money! If we stop buying these products, things will change. Use your "vote" wisely; *Buy more of what you want to see more of!!!*

And then there is all the confusing nutritional information out there: Fat is bad, fat is good, alcohol is ok, alcohol isn't ok... So, what do we need to do? We need to give the body what it needs (**nutrient richness**), and it's simple. There are two steps.

2 STEPS TO NUTRIENT RICHNESS:

1. **Hydration**: The amount of water we drink affects our moods, our cognitive abilities, and all our body processes. Staying well-hydrated is critical to improving and maintaining health.

2. **Whole Foods**: There is a balance of macronutrients (carbs, fats, proteins) and micronutrients (vitamins and minerals) in whole foods that are already figured out for us. Our bodies can easily process and absorb these nutrients.

1. Hydration: Studies have proven that when we're dehydrated, the first thing that is affected is our mood. We become irritable and angrier. Other studies demonstrate that drivers who were dehydrated while driving made as many mistakes as someone who is mildly alcohol-impaired. It obviously reduces our physical performance (by up to 10% vs. when we are optimally hydrated).

2. Whole Foods: Here, we need to focus not only on the Macronutrients (carbs, protein, fats) because everything HAS that, but *more importantly, the micronutrient requirements* (vitamins and minerals that come in perfect packages in perfect quantities in whole foods). Whole foods fulfill our nutritional needs, *and* they take up the space of refined foods that cause inflammation. I.E, they're fulfilling what the body needs AND protecting it from the harm of refined foods. We can even slow down the aging process by reducing oxidative stress. Red foods, berries, and leafy greens have antioxidants that slow down the aging process.

HOW DO WE DO ALL THIS?

First, Create Awareness! Then, stay hydrated and consume more whole foods. Simple, right?

1. CREATE AWARENESS:

What kind of hunger are you having?

* *Thirst*: If you stay hydrated throughout the day, your hunger will not be due to thirst. Drink up!

* *Nutritional Hunger*: Your body signals that it needs nutrients.

Low Blood Sugar: Has it been a while since you ate? Do you *need* food now?

* *Variety*: Make sure you are getting a variety of fruits, vegetables, and proteins from different sources to avoid food boredom.

* *Empty stomach*: This may feel unfamiliar at first if you are used to eating all day long. An empty stomach doesn't always *need* filling.

* *Emotional*: Are you looking to fill an emotional need? How else can you fill that need that doesn't require eating?

Listen to your internal dialogue:

What are your thoughts as you have a "craving"? What leads you to your choice? How do you feel after making a choice? How do you feel after the first bite? The second? Halfway through? After eating? 4 hours later? The next day? This can help us identify WHY we are choosing what we do and HOW that choice *actually* makes us feel. Pizza was a Friday night staple for me growing up, but now it always gives me a stomach ache, so today, I don't think it's worth it, and I just make other choices.

If you want to explore further: try an elimination diet to see how foods are affecting you. Is it a sensitivity, an intolerance, or an allergy? Check your symptom list created from your observations. (Consult your health care professional here if you have concerns.) Remove items for 3 weeks, then reintroduce 1 every 3 days, noting any changes.

2. HYDRATE WELL

Listen to your body. Sip all day instead of gulping down your daily quantity all at once. Carry a water bottle. *How much water do you need?* They say about 8 glasses per day. Some need more; some need less. Depends on your lifestyle, how much you sweat through exercise, climate, etc.

How do you know if you are optimally hydrated?

Follow your thirst. The body is designed to trigger thirst because water is *the* most important element that we need. Some people have been so habitually mildly dehydrated that they are out of touch with the body's signals. Your urine should be transparent, pale yellow...NOT dark yellow.

Habits to prevent mild dehydration:

* *Sipping* through the day is better than drinking half a litre at a time.

* *Carry a big bottle* of water everywhere you go.

* *Replenish electrolytes* for cell hydration. Drinking water and hydrating are 2 different things; you need electrolytes in order to use the water in your body. The water we drink goes to the bloodstream; we want to drive it into the cells of the body. Electrolytes manage this system and conduct electricity to open up or close the cells. With no electrolytes, water isn't absorbed from the bloodstream, so you can still experience symptoms of mild dehydration. We lose electrolytes during the day through exercise, sweating, and even at night through breathing. Therefore, we need to replenish first thing in the morning. Add a pinch of Himalayan or Celtic salt to your morning water (up to ¼ tsp to 1 Litre of water). It should NOT taste salty. If you have hypertension, always *check with your doctor* first (this amount generally should not affect your blood pressure).

3. CONSUME MORE WHOLE FOODS

Eat 80% whole foods. *Bonus:* eat foods high in antioxidants. Cells in the body convert food energy into physical energy using

64

mitochondria and oxygen. This energy is found in the form of adenosine triphosphate (ATP). This energy conversion process creates oxidative stress, an imbalance of free radicals and antioxidants in the body, which can lead to cell and tissue damage. Oxidative stress occurs naturally and plays a part in aging. Foods with antioxidants protect you from *too much* oxidative stress, and this supports a slower aging process.

Foods high in antioxidants:

* Berries (raspberries, blueberries, etc.) frozen is ok too
* Leafy greens (spinach, cabbage, lettuce, etc.)
* Red foods (beetroot, red bell pepper, etc.)

Use the *behavioural model*; choose the easiest way to meet this goal. Some of us aren't used to preparing our meals. Making complicated recipes with lots of spices may be a big leap to start. Use *Zero Resistant habits*; make it easy! Start with a few basic meals that give you what you need, and from there, you can elaborate.

Add these **3 easy recipes** to your diet to increase your fruit and vegetable intake. These recipes give us basic nutrition. One is a raw recipe, and two are cooked. They only take between 5 and 30 minutes from fridge to table.

I.   Staying Young Smoothie:

Put all items in your blender for a few minutes until you reach desired consistency. I have a Vitamix that is super speedy, but there is an order of ingredients for layering you need to follow. Check your machine. Choose items from the 4 categories on the left. Add options in the right category if desired.

BERRIES X1-2	EXTRAS:
BRIGHT RED X1 Beetroot Pomegranate Watermelon Grapefruit Red grapes	*CREAMINESS* Frozen cauliflower Ice
LEAFY GREENS X1 Spinach Kale	*SPICES* Cinnamon Clove

Collard greens	Ginger
LIQUID Water Plant milk	*ENERGY BOOST* Green tea Black tea Cacao
	FAT BOOST Pecans Sunflower seeds Chia seeds
	CARB BOOST Oats
	PROTEIN BOOST Whey Vegan Blend

II.　　**WholeBowls:** (15-minute prep, 15-minute cook time)
This is a great recipe to help you get all the nutrients you need in one bowl. It provides variety by having cooked and raw foods combined.

* First, cook what needs to be oven cooked. (eg. complex carbs like roasting the sweet potato because it takes the longest.) You can season with a spray of avocado oil, salt, and pepper. Mix with fingers and place in the oven for 15 min at 200 degrees.

* Second, use your stovetop to fry pan proteins, like chicken. Season to taste (e.g., s/p, garlic, cayenne, rosemary.) Cook protein for 5 min, then add the veggies after. I don't add oil *when* I cook. I will add it *later* for seasoning. Add more seasonings to the veggies. Lower heat to med.

* Next, take the oven foods out. Start preparing the WholeBowl with a bed of greens as the base. Add the raw veggies. For example, put sprouts on one side, tomatoes, pickles, and sweet potatoes, then dump the frypan foods on top.

* Add your healthy fats and drizzle olive oil or dressing on top if you like.

* The proportions are: 10% base, 20% veggies, 20% protein, 20% complex carbs, 10% healthy fats, 20% from the category on the right (fruit, microbiome treat, and dressing.)

BASE x1	EXTRAS:

Leafy Green	
Spinach	
Kale	
Rockets	
Lettuce	
VEGGIES x3	
Broccoli	
Cauliflower	
Zucchini	
Carrots	
Tomatoes	
Capsicum	
Mushrooms	
PROTEIN	*DRESSING*
x1 Chicken, Fish, Beef, Eggs	Olive Oil
X2 Tofu,Tempeh,Seitan,Legumes,	Lemon
Beans, Quinoa	Balsamic Vinegar
COMPLEX CARBS x1	*FRUIT*
Sweet potato	Berries
Peas	Mango
Corn	Apple
Parsnips	Pineapple
Brown Rice	Papaya
Buckwheat	
Millet	
HEALTHY FATS X1	*MICROBIOME TREAT*
Avocado	Sauerkraut
Nuts	Kimchi
Seeds	Pickles
Olive Oil	Apple Cider Vinegar
Coconut Oil	
Tahini	

III.   **HeroSoup**: Cooked foods, leftover vegetable parts (10 min prep, 30 min cook time).

A great way to use your remaining vegetable debris. A meal where you can have anything you wouldn't have raw. It gives us many micronutrients in one go that are easy to digest and very filling.

* Choose your favourite vegetables for the soup. Cut them all up and put them in a pot. Adding cauliflower will make it creamy. Add all your vegetable leftovers from the week. You can use all the vegetable parts.

For example, if you use squash, you can add peel and seeds, carrot or zucchini peels, etc. Use vegetables of all different colours. Fill the pot about ¾ from the top.

* Add half a pot of water.

* Add seasonings (s/p, ginger, saffron… whatever you like.)

* Cover and bring to a boil.

* Then reduce heat to med for about 20-30 min…poke veggies with a fork to see if they're soft and ready to blend.

* Put it all in the blender, especially the water. You can adjust the water amount…Less water makes it even creamier.

* Now, you're ready to eat.

HeroSoup can be kept in the fridge for a couple of days, or you can freeze it for later. If you make it very creamy, it can be a dip. Or, if it's very, very creamy, it can even be a spread. Add seeds on top, or spices…dill? Play with your favourite ingredients!

DEEPEN YOUR AWARENESS:

What are your main sources of each macronutrient?
What is your most satisfying meal? What is its macronutrient composition?
What is your most calorie-dense meal? How do you feel after eating it?

Increase your nutrient-dense foods:

* Leafy greens
* Meats and legumes
* Nuts and seeds
* Fruits and vegetables
* Root vegetables

A note about variety:

We are meant to eat a variety of foods. Historically, it was based around the seasons and food availability. Throughout the year, we would eat a variety of seasonal plants, fruits, and vegetables; meat availability would change throughout the year. But as we ate a rotating variety of food, we would get all our nutrients in the cycle of the year:

In *Spring*, we would have seen increased proteins, green leafy vegetables, and lots of water. These nutrients would signal to our body that food is abundant, and we can release our winter fat storage. Certain foods have been programmed into our DNA to do certain things. When we eat lots of green veggies, our brain thinks it's spring, and it starts to burn fat. Want to release weight? Eat lots of dark greens!

In *Summer*, we would have seen decreased animal proteins, increased root vegetables, and occasional berries. In *Fall,* even less meat and more fruit (higher sugar availability). In *winter*...sometimes imposed fasting; threat of starvation.

We are so fortunate now that what we eat is no longer dictated by the seasons. Anything we want is available pretty much anytime we want it. But that can be dangerous as well. Many of us eat sugar every day, all day. This signals to your body that winter is coming...I.E. PUT ON EXTRA WEIGHT. And we do, continually, without going through the cycle of gaining a bit for "winter" and losing it again in "spring". We just keep packing it on, new weight on top of the old weight. Winter is ALWAYS coming! Not a healthy state of things. We need to cycle this weight off and on. If you eat low sugar and lots of green vegetables, you will signal to your body that it's time to drop excess weight. So...**Think about eliminating sources of added sugars.**

It is also worth mentioning the effect of your environment. Does yours mesh with your food goals? You can design your home environment in ways that promote healthier choices. A technique I learned from *Ronan Diego de Oliveira,* called ***Adjust and Adios***, is helpful. You *adjust*: *promote* foods you want to eat (make them visible, like a bowl of fruit on the counter) and *demote* foods you don't want to eat often (make them invisible, like putting them in high cupboards or at the back of the shelf). Then you eliminate, say *Adios* to, foods that are on your "Not right now" list.

Decide your rules:

What is now below your level of acceptability? Create a grid; this is mine. Build yours according to your goals.

My Essential foods list:	My Acceptable/Optional foods list (useful but not necessary)
Water	
Leafy vegetable	Brown/wild rice
Nuts	Sweet potatoes
(Fruit, root veggies)	Avocado
Pinch of Himalayan salt	Almond milk
My Occasional Foods list:	**My Never Foods list:**
Tomatoes	Refined sugars,
Bell Peppers	Artificial sweeteners, colours, flavours,
Squash	chemical additives
Zucchini	Deep-fried foods / GMOs
Grains (corn, oats)	Processed foods
	Grains (wheat)
	Dairy
	Corner store chocolate
My rare foods list:	
Potatoes	
Honey	
Caffeine	
Really good quality chocolate	

Sometimes "forever" is daunting. Try saying, "I won't have this food right now" vs. "never". Create your boundaries and give yourself a break occasionally. I use **ratios**. 6:1 or 10:1 or 28:2 etc. Six days of healthy eating and one day to have something outside normal limits. Or ten days and one day, or 28 and 2 if I'm needing it. This helps keep me in check rather than letting a "slip" take me right off-track long term. I plan special events in my calendar and adjust my ratios. If I am going to have pancakes with a friend on Sunday, I don't have another "occasional" food for another 6 days.

I also practice **intermittent fasting**. I built up my practice from 12 to 16 hours, where I comfortably sit now. Your body needs to cycle through all its processing systems. Daytime is for adding fuel to our body and exercise, so we are ready for fight or flight needs. At night, we need to give our systems a rest, literally, so we can rest and digest and absorb the nutrients we consume during the day. This practice can be extremely helpful during menopausal phases. Look into it more if you are interested. There are several types: water fasting, green fasting, live food fasting, multiday fasting, and cleanses. As with everything else, do your research before you start anything. Remember to start slow and scale up.

A last important note: You should never allow yourself to get hungry. If we are hungry too long, our body thinks it is winter, and it turns everything into stored fat. It thinks it's starvation time. Eating nothing can make you gain weight. So...eat. But eat wisely. Drink lots of water, and munch on raw veggies.

YOUR TURN: Homework Time

Look at the areas of Nutrient Richness skills; where is your main opportunity (Building awareness, improving hydration, consuming more whole foods)? Choose ONE thing you will do this week to strengthen your Nutrient Rich toolbox. If you have a level one practice already, try level two or three.

Action steps/habit building

Level One:

* Listen to your body: which of the 6 hungers are you feeling?

* Listen to your internal dialogue: how does what you eat make you feel?

* Create a space for reflection at one meal of the day (more on this in another chapter)

Level Two:

* Follow the 2 Steps to nutrient richness.

* Follow the 80% whole foods rule.

* Create your "what's acceptable" grid, your "rules".

* Adopt recipes:
    * Staying Young Smoothie

* WholeBowls
* Herosoup

Level Three:

* Look at your macronutrient design. What is the best ratio for you?

* Increase your nutrient-rich foods. Try new fruits or vegetables. Experiment. Enjoy. Expand your recipes.

* Look into intermittent fasting.

* Refine your recipes for macronutrient and micronutrient design; create a repertoire of 3 master meals for breakfast, 3 for lunch and 3 for dinner.

Tips for cravings:

* Drink water and wait 10 minutes.
* Practice breathing exercises.
* Take a brisk 20-minute walk.
* Reach out to your support community.
* Keep checking your food pangs of hunger and internal dialogue.
* Anticipate and Plan: set limits, prep snacks, packs meals/snacks.

WHAT'S NEXT?

Phew! I warned you it was A LOT!

It IS a LOT! I know. But it can be done. Address changes first in the areas you feel will yield the best results. Take baby steps. Remember, changing too much too fast is NOT sustainable. You can always add more when you can maintain and are ready to scale up.

When you are ready, there is even more… I'm so passionate about this topic that I want to give you so much more. **But please *don't*** *look yet* *if you're feeling overwhelmed* already. Wait till you have mastered the basics before you start the ***advanced studies*** *section.*

I adopted all of these strategies step by step, as well as the advanced studies list, and virtually eliminated everything on my physical symptom list. All the adjustments in nutritional habits literally melted off any excess weight bringing me back to a healthy BMI without once counting calories.

I now have:

More mental clarity
Better memory
More energy, especially in the afternoons and evenings
More flexibility and fluid movements
Deeper sleep
Elimination of headaches
Elimination of arthritic pain
Clear airways and zero wheezing
Elimination of skin rashes
Elimination of respiratory and sinus congestion
Eliminated colds, flu and infections
Stronger muscles
Stronger hair and nails

I have a process to avoid self-sabotage and a get backup strategy for when I slip.

All of this combined to make a huge impact on my transformation. My body is **regulated** to a state of health as a consequence.

"If you can't fly then run, if you can't run then walk,
if you can't walk then crawl,
but whatever you do you have to keep moving forward."
Martin Luther King Jr.

You GOT THIS!

And now that we've slept well, gotten moving, gotten outside, and had something to eat, next we get quiet...

PROTECT THE BODY FROM HARM:

There is a difference between acute inflammation, which can be good for the body and promotes healing, and chronic inflammation. We are meant to be able to recover from acute inflammation, like from an injury. Cycle through and recover. Give the body what it needs, and it knows how to heal itself. But chronic inflammation is highly dangerous. It doesn't go away, and the effects are cumulative. It can cause:

* Xenobiotics
* Disturbed sleep
* Isolation
* Chronic stress
* Gut dysbiosis
* Obesity
* Physical inactivity
* Chronic infections

Everything is interconnected. Obesity means more visceral fat around the organs. This visceral fat is where toxins are stored. Any time this fat is turned into energy, we release the toxins into our organs and immune system. Diet is generally the root cause of obesity, and that means lifestyle changes to tackle it. We need to focus on reducing chronic inflammation. Physical movement and quality sleep also contribute to reducing systemic inflammation. Keep up those new habits!

Part of protecting the body from harm also includes:

RESTORING INSULIN RESISTANCE & ELIMINATING HIGH-GRADE INFLAMMATION

We are flooding our systems with sugar all day, every day, with all the processed foods we eat. I know, I keep on about sugar, but... Much of the world's population is insulin resistant now. Almost ALL processed

74

foods have sugar added. Check the labels carefully. If it isn't whole food and you didn't make it from scratch using whole foods...it likely has sugar. The worst offenders are the *added sugars and indulgent grains*.

Added Sugars and Indulgent Grains:

What is the correlation between sugar and inflammation? For that, we need to understand how the body uses sugar...and what happens when we put more into our systems.

When we eat carbs, our body turns them into glucose (sugar) which is the main source of fuel that our body uses. There is always some sugar running through our bloodstream. Normally we have about 4g of glucose in our bloodstream and cannot keep more than that. To avoid too much sugar in the bloodstream, we have a pancreas that produces the hormone insulin. This takes the sugar and stores it in the liver or the muscle masses or in your fat cells, so it doesn't harm the major arteries.

When we have too much sugar intake (e.g., constant sugar load in every meal) and insulin is being produced all the time, eventually, our cells become resistant to insulin, and our body will require more to allow the cells to absorb sugar. Insulin resistance can develop over the years if this process keeps occurring.

Insulin resistance is not only an inflammatory agent on its own, but all the cells of the immune system (24 different types like T cells, B cells, neutrophils, macrophages, etc.) are mediated by insulin. If the body becomes resistant, then the operation of the *immune system* is off balance. Insulin resistance can also lead to *obesity and diabetes* and a cascade of events in the body. We need to cut the problem from the root by *reducing our sugar consumption*.

The recurring consumption of sugar operates in our brains and is habit-building. A high amount of sugar increases the release of dopamine (pleasure) in our brains. We are hardwired to repeat the habits that reward us chemically. It is a DNA design to guarantee our survival. Ancestrally, sugar helped us put on fat to survive the winter. But now..."winter" is always coming. We need to cycle out of "winter". If we reduce our consumption, we lower the craving and reduce the habit.

Additionally, *gut microbiomes* are disrupted by too much sugar. Bad bacteria then start growing in the wrong places in your gut, killing the good bacteria that are digesting your food. It also starts to impair the gut walls. These are meant to allow nutrients to come inside and keep harmful things outside, but if that wall is broken, harmful things enter our bloodstream, which gives signals to our immune system...which then generates more inflammation. You see the cycle?

There can even be a disruption to our **sex hormones** : for men, high concentrations of sugar decrease testosterone (one study showed 75g of sugar in a single meal can decrease levels by 35% for 2 hours); for women, it can increase testosterone production even to the point of stopping ovulation.

How can we remove the root causes of potential harm? Where should we focus? We start with those things that create most of the impact. Not all sugars and grains are "bad". We want to remove *added sugars and indulgent grains*. Where do we find these? Let's look at the types of sugars and grains.

TYPES OF SUGARS

* Naturally occurring: Natural sugars in fruits and vegetables, roots. These do not cause the majority of harm or damage, so we *do not focus on removing them right now* (unless you have diabetes or other medical concerns)

* Avoid Added sugars: There are 65 different names for sugar because food manufacturers know we are on the lookout for sugar on labels, and they try to disguise it. This is the biggest area of added sugars in our diets. Read labels.

* Avoid Sugary beverages: These include pop, flavoured specialty coffees, and juice. Did you know that one bottle of OJ has 13 oranges, *and* their sugars and fibre are removed, which decreases the rate of absorption of that sugar in our bodies? It's like having 13 oranges with no benefit...just lots of sugar.

TYPES OF GRAINS

* Whole grains: Barley, oatmeal, brown rice, buckwheat, etc.

* Refined grains: (Refined means there's only part of the grain used; it goes through an industrial process) These include staples like white rice, pasta, and bread. These may be causing some harm, but *indulgent grains* are causing the MOST harm when they are present in our daily routines. So, focus there first.

* Avoid Indulgent grains: Cookies, donuts, cakes, waffles, muffins, pizza, etc. These are not only refined grain devoid of nutrition, but they also contain added sugars and trans fats. If we stop eating these, it removes a huge cluster of things that are causing the most harm.

Let's start with sugar. *How can we remove sugar from our daily consumption?* First need to know where you're at.

WHERE ARE YOU AT WITH SUGAR CONSUMPTION?

Identify and check labels of what you eat and drink during the day for 2 days. Check labels. Find your main sources.

	FREE Of added sugars or indulgent grains	MINOR < 6g for women < 9g for men	MAJOR > 6g for women > 9g for men
MEALS * Breakfast * Lunch * Dinner			
DRINKS * Coffee/tea * Juice * Pop * Alcohol			
SNACKS * Morning * Afternoon * Evening			
Any surprising foods?			

Pay most of your attention and efforts to major appearances first, then make adjustments in your minor category. Did you find any foods that surprised you that had added sugar? Lots of food has added salt, sugar, and fat because the combination makes fireworks in our brains, and the impulse is to eat MORE.

LETTING GO: 2 ways...

A) Gradual:
For people who have most of their issues in the minor category and just need to make a few adjustments in their day.)

STRATEGIES

* Replace with complex carbs, which helps to avoid cravings, especially in the beginning.

* Replace beverages.

* B-MAP for major appearances (go back to behavioral design models from previous lessons to design new habits)

* Remove items from your home.

* Plan snacks.

* Lastly, remove sweeteners if you're having cravings (even zero-calorie sweeteners can trigger insulin release)

B) Cold Turkey (if there are major occurrences):
For people who have mostly major category issues. This may seem counterintuitive, but it may take a long time to move to no sugar through a gradual approach because there is a lot of habit-building involved and many triggers for relapse. It may be easier to go cold turkey on major occurrences.

* Have nothing sweet for 3 days (even fruit or root veggies because we are cutting the sweet taste from our tongues to rebuild taste buds). Your tongue can become numb from too much sugar. Taste buds need time to grow back.
* Reintroduce fruit and root vegetables slowly.

SIX OTHER THINGS TO LET GO OF:

A.   **Vegetable oils**: inflammatory fats: avoid the big 4 CSRP
     C= canola, cotton seed, corn oils
     S= soybean, sunflower, safflower oil
     R= rapeseed oil, rice bran oil
     P= palm oil

Instead, use olive, flax seed, avocado, hemp or coconut oil. Refine recipes with good oils, replace snack ingredients/new ideas, prep your own ready-to-eat meals in advance, cook more at home, or request changes in restaurants. Think about it...A restaurant menu is just a badly organized list of ingredients...be brave...be THAT person! Ask for what you want!!

B)   **Trans fats**: Estimated to be responsible for 20% of heart attacks. They're in 100% of crackers, 90% of cookies, cakes, pies, microwave popcorn, 80% of frozen meals, non-dairy creamers, and restaurant meals (fried chicken, fries, frying oils).

Not all oils and fats are good for you. The *main source of inflammation* comes through the food manufacturing process. (Check out the TV show *How It's Made: Canola Oil*) Large amounts of vitamins and fibers are removed, and chemical compounds are added that our bodies cannot digest. These products are mainly chemicals with a little bit of plant oil. Our body sees these as invaders (not food) and starts to fight them.

Also, Polyunsaturated fats: PUFA... We need Omega 3 (antioxidants) & Omega 6 (nuts, seeds). Whole foods have a natural balance of each that our bodies can tolerate. But if we add large amounts of Omega 6 (which is a pro-inflammatory, unstable molecule that, when it reacts with oxygen, creates a free radical cascade of more inflammation) through these oils, and we lack Omega 3, then our bodies are exposed to a lot of inflammation without the by-product to mitigate it.

We need *some* Omega 6 to generate some level of inflammation because this is our healing process and is good for our bodies, but too much creates problems. When our immune system needs to fight a virus, bacteria, or anything else, it uses energy stored through fat cells. If the cells have only Omega 6, it's like trying to put out a fire with gasoline. It just creates more problems.

C) **Grain-fed saturated fats**: Grain-fed animals store unhealthy fats and Omega 6s, especially those that have a single-compartment stomach, like chickens and pigs.

Avoid fatty cuts. When you feed grains to animals, they store unhealthy fats and Omega 6s just like we do.

Monogastric Animals: (pigs, poultry) Eating mammals with single-compartment stomachs adds more Omega 6s. It remains stored in their fat calls. Avoid fatty cuts of monogastric animals. It can take up to 3 years to clear from our body...

Ruminant Animals: (cattle, sheep, goats, deer) are usually fed with low-quality grains full of pollutants. Although they turn PUFA into saturated fats, they still carry a lot of toxins due to the low-quality grains they are fed. Try to avoid these as well.

STRATEGIES

* Cooking: Try olive oil, coconut oil, avocado oil, flax oil, hemp oil (all of these are either high in monounsaturated fat or saturated fat from a great source)

* Dressings: Try replacing ingredients (lemon, olive oil, herbs, spices)

* Snacks: New ideas, replace ingredients

* Ready to eat: Plan in advance / make your own. When we are "starving" with no plan, our food choice options become "more liberal/acceptable". Don't get too hungry, and plan in advance.

* Eating out: Request substitutions...(a menu is just a badly organized list of ingredients...be that person!) or prioritize COOKING more...build new habit ☺

* Meats: Opt for lean cuts; grass-fed fat (tallow and suet from a butcher); grass-fed and finished meat (minced chuck roast is a cheaper option).

    D)   **Tobacco**: (contributes to xenobiotics, and...you know the rest)

    The last 2 things were explored in the Sound Sleep chapter:

E)   Sleep disruptors

F)   Blue light

ELIMINATING ENDOCRINE DISRUPTORS:

Our environment has many toxins that cause harm to our bodies. Sites like **EWG.org** list disruptors to watch out for and even rate products for their level of toxic ingredients. Categories like "Food Scores, Skin Deep, Tap Water, and EWG verified products" can be helpful in identifying things to avoid. The areas of most impact in keeping us healthy here include:

1. Robust detoxing (eat fibre, sweat, use a sauna, exercise)
2. Large exposure sources (eat organic produce, grass-fed meats, free-range chicken, wild-caught fish)
3. Environmental sources (plastics, cosmetics, fragrances)
   Do consider tackling these issues as well.

OTHER considerations:

If you are looking at a *weight loss goal*, there are 2 general models:

* CICO (Calories In Calories Out model): There are some inherent flaws in this system. Manufacturers have a 20% margin of error in labeling calories of processed foods. Calorie burn rates differ from person to person based on age, activity level, etc. Many factors can affect this. However, it can be useful as a loose focus to monitor calories consumed. It must be pointed out that not all calories are designed equally. An apple at 80 calories provides much more than a small bag of chips for 80 calories.

So, it obviously isn't JUST calories we need. They need to be the *right* calories to help our bodies. You can use apps like **TDEEcalculator.net** (total daily energy expenditure) and calculate your optimal caloric intake based on your goals. Then you can design master meals around your needs. It's all a bit complicated for the scope of this book, but it can be helpful for some people. There are apps like **Chronometer** that can track micronutrients etc. as well if you want to go deep.

* CIM (The Carbohydrate Insulin Model): This idea is that weight gain is promoted by a high carbohydrate, high sugar diet, i.e., high levels of insulin. It focuses on proteins and vegetables as a base. This system doesn't work for everyone's body. For me, it made a huge difference. I didn't ever have to count calories, and I was never hungry.

You need to find the system that works for you. I hate counting calories and love veggies, so it was a better fit for me to try the CIM. And my body responded very well. I also credit my lost weight from eliminating dairy products from my diet and drastically reducing my grain intake. I'll tell you why I did that.

It is my "Side note", and you may not like it. I don't eat grains often, and now I *never* have dairy products because of things I learned and because of how my body reacts. I could say a whole lot more here, but it would be the length of another book... I'll just say this:

<u>Milk</u> is for babies.

I have learned some ghastly things about milk that drove me right off it. And I was a FANATIC about milk. I was one of those who grabbed the carton from the fridge and drank straight from it.

Did you know the countries with the highest milk consumption in the world are also the countries with the highest rates of osteoporosis? Hmmmm....

Above and beyond that, cow's milk is designed to grow a baby cow to 1000 pounds in a year. Our increased rates of consumption, propagated by marketing, have correlated with an increasing rise in obesity. Hmmm....

And finally, are you aware that milk contains an "acceptable level of puss" from mastitis in cows? And the level is constantly rising. Ewwwww....

Grains are for birds.

Grains have a protective coating that is ever-evolving so that they will remain undigested and transported through elimination. This coating irritates our systems. There is actually nothing we *need* nutritionally from grains. As we moved from being hunters and gatherers and learned to stay in one place and catch and grow food, grains became a way of preventing starvation in lean and vulnerable times. It was not intended to become the staple that it is now.

Did you know that Kellogg's hired a dietitian in 1924 to design the 4 food groups (first of all... 4 food groups? Sounds ridiculous even to say it)? Funny how that governmentally endorsed "Food group" pyramid contained a recommendation for a whopping 6-11 servings of grain! More than any other food group. And to boot, Kellogg's created breakfast cereals with loads of sugar; often, it's the number 2 ingredient.

You get the idea. IMHO, neither milk nor grains are people food... LOL. If you feel daring, I encourage you to try an elimination diet to see what effects these foods are having on *your* system. Everyone is different. My system reacts poorly to both.

I wish you all the awareness and empowerment to find your best nutritional fit!

CHAPTER 7

JUST SAY... Ohmmmm...

Week 5: Inner Stillness

Creating Inner Stillness is important! Why? Well, because life is chaotic! I know, I know! You don't have time...you're too stressed for any inner stillness crap! And that's exactly the point.

Think about this: Our ancestors had to deal with a stressful event once in a while...the lion approaches on occasion. But us? Our lifestyles are full of unpredictability and uncertainty, leading us to feel a lack of control. The traffic in the morning making you late, the lineup that's taking too long, the dirty look from a co-worker, the homework you didn't help your child with...what will "they" think of me?

Many of these events trigger a biological interpretation...a threat to our sense of "belonging". Ancestrally, being an outcast from the tribe meant certain death. Any threat that may cause "outcast" is dangerous...

This stimulates a **mammalian stress response** and a cascade of physiological events. Cortisol and adrenaline are released, and blood goes from the prefrontal cortex (logical decision-making) to the amygdala (fear and anxiety), which creates an urge to ACT (fight or flight).

We encode a traumatic response: *increase heart rate to provide more energy*, *immune cells stop repairing* and gather on the skin to protect from potential injury as that it the most likely spot for potential injury, energy for *digestion shuts down*, the liver releases *sugar to the blood* for energy to run (flight), blood goes to the arms, and legs ready to kick and punch (fight). Short-term memory goes (you don't need to remember where your PJs are when the lion approaches. Instead, the event is coded into long-term memory as "There is a threat is in THIS place at THIS time every Wednesday," etc., so that you remember not to be there at that time again). You become a momentary superhero to fight a predator or run from one. This process enabled us to survive.

Our stress response has served us well in strengthening our survival during unknown, unpredictable, stressful situations and was manageable when stressors were far less common for our ancestors than it is for us on a daily basis. It was Acute Stress, which is good for us and promotes healing processes in the body. But in modern society, this cycle of recurrent stress is repeated throughout the course of a day, every day, every month, and every year...the cumulative effect creates a state of **Chronic Stress.**

WHY IS THAT SO IMPORTANT? It causes:

* Weight gain
* Diabetes
* Heart disease
* Ulcers
* Infertility
* Immune dysfunction
* Mood & brain disorders
* Perceiving stress as dangerous raises our cortisol levels

Rates of anxiety are increasing world-wide. And the cascading health consequences of chronic stress are debilitating us. *The purpose of developing your inner stillness is to increase your resilience to stress!* Or *everything* else starts to shut down.... It has happened to me several times.

More importantly, we need to access skills of inner stillness to engage and promote healing states in our bodies. Isn't that why you are here reading?

HOW DO WE DO ALL THIS?

There are 3 components to developing **Inner Stillness:**

1) *Increase Your Resilience to Stress (a skill that requires practice and can grow in proficiency)*
2) *Reduce Your Sources of Stress* (harder, requires self-examination)

3) *Respond Skillfully to Stress* (is a practice, a routine that can be built)

If we start by addressing these three components of inner stillness, we will make a massive difference to your physiological and mental health. We need to spend more time in the Rest and Digest state so we can benefit from the nutrients we consume and so our bodies can efficiently do what they need to do when they need to do it.

So, let's start with:

INCREASING YOUR RESILIENCE TO STRESS:

* Connect to and strengthen your *social network*. It is literally the most important thing you can do for your overall resilience and health. (We will look at this more in a further chapter). Where do you spend most of your time? What are your interests and hobbies? If you do nothing else…do this! It's a BIG one!

* Physiologically speaking, and very, very briefly at that (as these topics are covered much more extensively in a previous chapter):
We need to Exercise: it sends stress-reducing hormones through your system.
We need to Eat well: increased fish oil and magnesium.
We need to Reduce stimulants: caffeine, etc.

Now let's go inward. ***Mindfulness practices:***

* Most importantly, here is developing an *attitude of GRATITUDE*!

"The more you are in a state of gratitude,
the more you will attract things to be grateful for"
Walt Disney

You know it, too; it is not a new idea. Name 5 things you are grateful for each day. This daily practice shifts your whole reality. Ever heard the expression… *"When you change what you're looking at, what you're looking at changes"*?   We all know the benefits but…***are you*** actually putting in the effort to thank the universe for the gifts you have been given? It's a fantastic way to start!!!

* Next, create moments of introspection and solitude in your day just for you. Even just 5-10 minutes. What will you do?

A 10-minute gaze out a window
A walk in the park
A hot cup of tea in a beautiful mug
Calming music break
Watching a candle flame
Listening to the birds
Sitting by a babbling brook
Doodling with all your favourite colours
Reading of few pages of an inspiring book
What else appeals to you?

And ....now...let's talk about...

* Meditation = The Four-Letter Word (here it is... I *DID* warn you...)

I feel some of you rolling your eyes, and mine used to as well. "I don't have time, and it never works..." Quite frankly, I don't even really like that term: "meditation". I admit it triggers me a bit to my past failures with adopting the practice. I'm not a sit-still-and-be-quiet kind of gal. "Meditation is for monks," I used to say.

I grew up in the 70s and 80s, and "altered states" was becoming popular. I strove to find those altered states but had no idea what I was doing. I tried sitting quietly and emptying my mind...have you ever tried to do that? It's like saying, "Don't breathe." That never worked for me.

I tried candles and music and dabbled in automatic writing. But I just couldn't do it. I even made poor choices as a young person trying to access these states using...well, unwise substance choices. But that didn't get me what I was after either...it just made me stupid or paranoid. But recently, I found something that FINALLY made sense.

There is a difference between *passive meditation* (mindfulness, quieting the mind, focusing on the breath) and *active meditation* (where you turn problems into projects). THIS resonated...

I needed to know *what* to access, *how* to access it, and *why* I was accessing it. "Altered States," I learned, was really just changing my brain wave frequency, slowing it down. It meant different levels of consciousness. Not only that, but I could have a purpose for "meditation"...beyond just sitting quietly waiting for the universe to unfold and enlighten me.

"We have, undoubtedly, certain finer fibers that enable
us to perceive truths when logical deduction,
or any other willful effort of the brain, is futile."
Nikola Tesla

70% of the world's cultures have polyphasic awareness, yet Western societies have abandoned this skill and have come to focus solely on a monophasic state of awareness. We have learned to be in one state most of the time and to value only that. Training your brain to become more polyphasic allows you to tap into "altered states" of mind. We live in a human body that *can move between different levels of consciousness.*

I learned more about the states of consciousness or different brain wave frequencies:

Gamma: 21+ Hz not fully researched yet
Beta: 14–21 Hz   outer conscious level; waking state
Alpha: 7–14 Hz   inner conscious level; meditation, ESP, intuition, creativity
Theta: 4–7 Hz deep meditation; intuition, strong psychic abilities
Delta: 1–4 Hz unconscious level; sleep state; higher intelligence, problem-solving

Although we can learn to use other levels for different purposes, for the points of our discussion, here, I will focus on the Alpha level of consciousness, how to access it and its benefits.

Generally, there are 4 ways to access Alpha:

Neurotraining: which is expensive and exclusive

Plant medicine: for which, you need an expert and guidance

Breathe work: which takes practice and time

Meditation: which is the easiest and cheapest way to access Alpha by learning to slow down your brain wave frequency (this can be measured on an EEG)

When we go beyond passive meditations to ACTIVE meditation (meditation with a specific purpose, turning problems into projects), we access different states to shift reality towards our vision. This thought has now become more mainstream. "Flow states" are based around this idea.

This made more sense to me; it was what I was looking to understand. I learned *what* to access, *how* to access it, and *why* I was accessing it. I learned to slow my brain wave frequency down to allow me to work on "projects" (goals, visions, and especially healing). I learned a 40-day technique to train my brain in accessing an Alpha state of consciousness, which I'll include instructions for later.

I realised that when we occupy space for inner stillness, we are in an environment where the body heals itself. Just like sleep is the environment where our body repairs and grows, active meditation is the environment for the body to heal itself.

I was fortunate enough to study under *Vishen Lakhiani* to learn and become certified in teaching the **Silva UltraMind Method** *for healing the body*. It was a revolutionary moment for me! It was so similar to things I had been taught as a child by my grandma (in secret...we did not talk about these things with others way back then...it was the 70s). This was home for me...

If you haven't heard of *Jose Silva*, designer of the **Ultramind Method**, I urge you to look up his story. His technique is now used by some of the most famous athletes and business gurus, regular folks like you and me, and has been spreading worldwide for decades. He designed a specific script to trigger the brain for healing. It uses a *"3 Scenes"* approach to turn problems into projects that the brain works out. By focusing on the pain, the action, and the effects of the result, you learn to program your brain to enlist alternate strategies you hadn't thought of to bring about the vision you seek. Your body even experiences the healing process you are practicing envisioning AS you practice.

I further became certified in teaching *Vishen Lakhiani's* **6-Phase Meditation technique,** a complete meditation regime that focuses on the NOW and the FUTURE.

Both these programs are, unfortunately, too comprehensive to explain in a book, but I have practiced it myself and taught many, many others these techniques with amazing results!

And, If you're still doubting the power of the mind and how you can improve your health through these techniques, I encourage you to pick up the book **Mind Over Medicine: Scientific Proof That You Can Heal Yourself** by *Lissa Rankin, MD.* Just do it!!

Sometimes, during these inner stillness practices, things come up...resistance to something, an old belief or pattern that is holding you back. It can be a great time to examine what's helping you and what is hindering you.

With these practices, I have healed eczema, healed respiratory infections, eliminated chronic migraines, solved problems, resolved a conflict, grown my business, and developed new project ideas... Really, it's just an endless list of powerhouse results.

So, are you ready to embark on one of the most powerful habit journeys of this book? Let's get to work...

HOW DO WE PLAN ALL THIS?

1. INCREASE RESILIENCE TO STRESS:

A) *Assess your social network:*

* Identify your "3 or more" people that you can count on for joy and support. Plan ONE social activity (a phone call, a visit, a walk, a video chat, a tai chi class)...anything that makes you happy and is DOABLE for this week. We will cover this topic in greater detail in the

next chapter as it is a core element of the 7 Habits. Employing your social support network is the main factor (having 3 or more friends you can count on).

* Here's the hard one! Are there relationships that are causing stress that you can scale down or let go of?

B) *Adopt mindfulness practices:*

There are infinite choices here, depending on your personal preferences. Sit quietly and gaze out a window, go for a brisk solo walk, read a few pages of an inspiring book, write 5 gratitudes... any activities that resonate. All you need to do is to make space in your daily routine for 10-15 minutes of introspection and appreciation.

You can also use: *Mindfulness-Based Stress Reduction* **MBSR techniques** such as labeling sensations/triggers, gratitude practices focusing on positives, managing physiological elements like exercise and caffeine, and increasing fish oil/Omega 3 fatty acids & magnesium.

This 40-day process trains your brain to get into the Alpha state of consciousness. You can even play "**Alpha beats**" (search on YouTube) to help your brain calibrate to the correct speed.

40-DAY TECHNIQUE TO ACCESS ALPHA:

Accessing Alpha: you are already in alpha in the first 5 minutes after waking up. This is the best time to tune in to train the mind and practice. You don't need to clear your mind; the goal is just to relax and tune in to Alpha.

Day 1-10: Sit upright, count gently from 100 to 1. This will take 3-5 minutes. You will be in Alpha.

Day 11-20: Sit upright, count from 50 to 1. This will take 2 minutes. You will be in Alpha.

Day 21-30: Sit upright, count from 20 to 1. You will be in Alpha.

Day 31-40: Sit upright, count from 10 to 1. You will be in Alpha.
Day 41 onwards: Sit upright, count from 5 to 1 anytime you want to be in Alpha.

2. REDUCE SOURCES OF STRESS:

Assess your main sources of stress. Usually, the top 5 are:
* Relationships
* Work
* Loss
* Big Changes
* Illness

Review your goals: Are they causing you any stress? For each goal, ask yourself: Do I truly want it? Is it worth it? Can I outsource parts of the task?

List your main stressors: Are there any ongoing and regular sources of stress you can eliminate? Are there relationships you need to scale down or let go of?

Do you need to bring in more **self-care**? (Women are hard-wired to care for others during stressful times at their own expense. Evaluate your efforts here.)

Are you **avoiding processing** any stressful situations? Do you need to seek guidance or support here?

3) RESPOND SKILLFULLY TO STRESS:

Try breathing exercises from 1-3x per day or whenever you need calm. Manage your central nervous system through your breath by using the *4x7x8 technique:*

A) Breathe in deeply for a count of 4
B) Hold your breath for a count of 7
C) Exhale fully for a count of 8
D) Repeat 8 times

Or, try *alternate nostril breathing*

A) Cover the left nostril and breathe in through the right
B) Cover the right and breathe out through the left
C) Breathe in again through the left
D) Cover the left and exhale through the right
E) Repeat cycle 6x

Breathing through the diaphragm or deep breathing. We often use **"prey"** breathing (shallow and quiet so as not to be heard by predators; a needed skill prehistorically). Breathing deeply activates your parasympathetic nervous system and signals to your body that all is safe.

Exercise, eat well (including Omega3s, fish oil), reduce stimulants (caffeine, alcohol, tobacco).

AREAS FOR FURTHER STUDY if you're interested:

* Silva UltraMind Method – get taught by a certified instructor
* 6-Phase Meditation – get taught by a certified instructor
* Book: *Altered States* by Daniel Goleman
* Book: *Stealing Fire* by Stephen Kotler
* Book: *Mind Over Medicine: Scientific Proof You Can Heal Yourself* by Lissa Rankin, M.D.

YOUR TURN: Homework Time

Look at the 3 areas of inner stillness skills; where is your main opportunity (increasing resilience, reducing sources, or responding skilfully)? Choose ONE thing you will do this week to strengthen your inner stillness toolbox. If you have a level one practice already, try a level two or three.

Action steps/habit building

Level One:

* Start the 4x7x8 breathing technique at least once a day or whenever you need inner calm. I do this religiously right before I go to sleep.

* Name 5 things you are grateful for each day. Write it down with a beautiful pen in a treasured journal. Make it special.

* Make space in your daily routine for 10 - 15 minutes of introspection and appreciation. Sit quietly and gaze out a window, go for a brisk solo walk, read a few pages of an inspiring book... any activities that resonate.

Level Two:

* Evaluate your stressors; do you have some tough choices to make? What is possible?

* Begin training your brain to access the Alpha state using the 40-day technique.

Level Three:

* Get trained in using the power of your mind for healing, whether it's healing relationships, solving work problems, manifesting goals, or healing the body. It is one of the most powerful things you can do for your health.

WHAT IS NEXT?

You know the drill. All this sounds simple, but it takes **practice.** Daily practice helps strengthen this skill. Address the area first that you feel will yield you the best results. Start with baby steps. Remember, changing too much too quickly is NOT sustainable. You can always add more when you are able to maintain and ready to scale up in this category. When you adopt level one practices, move on to level two and three as you are ready.

Speaking of people in our lives...up next week: **Your BFFs!**

CHAPTER 8

BESTIES!

Week 6: **Deep Connections**

I'm going to tell you something now that you'll probably want to kick me for...

Having deep social connections is the **NUMBER ONE MOST IMPORTANT** factor in your health and longevity! If you only focus on one thing... **do this**!!!

WHAAAAAAAT? WHY didn't I say that at the beginning? LOL

In working on our baseline of health and fitness, several new habits may have needed to be adopted. There was a need to focus on ourselves...to start by giving our body what it needs and protecting it from harm. Now, we focus on our social connections in life.

This isn't new; we know our social connections are important. I noticed this *need* was clearly amplified during our isolation through COVID 19. The movement to "work from home" left us even more isolated during workday periods. Advanced technology that allows us to stay in touch with others remotely has been the biggest blessing. But as we became accustomed to isolation and now as things open up, I notice now that we say we "value" socializing, but we do not "practice" it. Some of us had a hard time re-emerging from isolation. Are you now out and about seeing others like you did pre-COVID? Slowly, bit by bit, we are starting to open up and see other people in person. Which is fantastic!!

Our need to belong is embedded in our DNA. For our ancestors, to be cast out of the tribe meant certain death. The need to belong isn't a character trait...it's in our DNA as a survival skill. Threats to our tribe membership privileges are stressful, and you well know by now the harmful effects of stress.

Remember **Maslow's Hierarchy?** Once people's safety and physiological needs are met, they are driven to seek connection with other people (love and belonging). We crave it. If your need to **belong** is met, you may feel invincible...like you can conquer the world. Even my most (often self-proclaimed) "reclusive" friends and relatives have at least 3 deep connections in their lives.

I invite you to look up one of *Harvard* University's longest studies, the **"Very Happy People"** study, run by *Ed Diener and Martin Seligman*, spanning 80 years. It showed that our strong social connections are the only truly correlated factor in our happiness with a demonstrated, and remarkable, 0.7 correlation to happiness. This is a massive statistic in the scientific world.

The closeness of the relationships is what matters the most. Studies show you are 50% more likely to survive a dangerous illness if you have strong social bonds. You also have 39% less chance of heart disease, 32% less chance of stroke, and many other striking statistics...and this is regardless of other habits like smoking, alcohol consumption, obesity, and sedentary lifestyles.

In fact, the scientific evidence of this is mounting. Have you heard of the **Roseto Effect**? The phrase is based on a study of a close-knit community in Roseto, Pennsylvania, USA. Despite behavioural habits (like consumption of unfiltered cigar smoking, alcohol and soda pop, and high fried fat and meat-based diet), the community had nearly no heart attacks in the significantly high-risk group of men studied. Lower rates of heart disease were attributed to the lower stress rates of the community because of their close bonds.

It wasn't because they had special Italian DNA, because they didn't. It wasn't because they followed a Mediterranean diet because they didn't. It wasn't because they were non-smokers because they weren't. It wasn't because they didn't drink alcohol because they did. It wasn't because they didn't consume sugar because they did. It wasn't because of **any** factors other than their close bonds within the community. Google it if you're interested.

It doesn't even necessarily have to be a huge social network. The *National Institute of Aging* quantifies the "magic" number as at least 3 friends who care about you, and you can go to for support. I used to

96

have a huge social group. 100+ colleagues, some closer than others, a group of 20 to go out every Friday night, brunch friends, hiking friends, and family to visit.

During COVID-19, our connections with colleagues were challenged as we all briefly worked from home. When we returned to the building together, social interactions were discouraged for safety reasons. After 3 years...it became normal. Many of us even re-evaluated the quality of some of those friendships (as we all realised our time was precious and values shifted). Many friendships were let go. Not for reasons of conflict...just lack of reciprocal efforts. Priorities change. But...Our NEED for social connection does not. We just became a little more discerning about it, I think.

Today, as a midlife woman changing careers and starting new chapters, I have reorganized and reprioritized the relationships in life. My social circle is smaller, and I am no less happy than when it was huge! It surprized me, really. I've always been the social butterfly type... I loved having tons of friends and different experiences. But now, I am actually more content with a smaller circle of supporters in my corner. I can give those in my life the time and energy they deserve rather than giving whatever is left of me at the end. I've stopped putting so much effort into relationships that aren't reciprocal. I still feel fulfilled and am happier than ever.

Historically, our need for belonging was met by belonging to tribes, then by belonging to developing communities, then by belonging to institutions (often religious, military). The strength of these institutions is now waning...for better or for worse. I don't mean to engage you in a political discussion here. The point is that people are looking to fill the void of "not belonging" to something, and without the strength of these institutions drawing them in, they generally look to seek it out in the workplace.

Many people spend more time with coworkers than with family... Yet as the economic landscape has been forever changed by COVID, and as people increasingly want to work remotely for flexibility of childcare, travel, scheduling, and commuting costs. We are remaining more isolated.

Now, I've always been one to highly value my alone time due to my childhood upbringing. But my relative, who grew up in the same circumstance, despises alone time. Everyone responds differently. It's a balance. But I know I need people, and people need me. And while I do take time to recharge my batteries and spend time in inner stillness… I always go back to my people.

So, I will say it again: If you take nothing else from this book, please take this with you:

Your deep connection with other people is the biggest factor that will impact and improve your health and longevity and your overall happiness in life.

HOW DO WE DO THIS?

Going back to the **Data/studies from NIA** (National Institute of Aging) that asks questions to determine how long/well you are going to live, one of the critical questions asked is:

"Do you have at least **3** friends that care about you and you can reach out to?"

Do they support you when you are in need? DO you have a great time together? If so, FANTASTIC! YAY, YOU!!! Keep on trucking and nurturing those relationships *as if your life depended on them*… because it literally does!!! IF not, what can we do…? Let's look at 3 steps:

CLEAR THE GUTTER: It may seem counterproductive, but sometimes we need to clear the gutter first.

Do you have **any hard decisions** to make about those you let into your life? Are there any toxic relationships that can be *let go or scaled down*? Are you putting too much energy into unfulfilling relationships? Can your energy be put to better use?

Sometimes people come into our lives and leave our lives for a reason. It can take hindsight to see the reasons. But often, if the "purpose" of the connections is complete, the relationship will evaporate. It is a normal cycle of life. It can be hard to accept sometimes, but think: who do you want to give your energy to the most? I don't mean to sound cold here, but you only have so much time and energy.

ENHANCE CURRENT RELATIONSHIPS: Of those relationships you choose to keep, how can you enhance them?

* I often make phone calls when I go on my daily walk to connect with family or friends if we can't get together physically. Go ahead and do it cold...no appointment. See if we can change the social culture back to the days when you could just call someone rather than texting, "Can I call you today?"

* I walk every day. I invite friends to new locations once a week. Sometimes it's a short 20-minute walk to catch some Vitamin D and a chat. Other times it's a longer 90 min walk through a local trail.

* I have standing "dates" with a bestie at the end of the week.

* I joined a weekly local Tai Chi class, and our ritual is Chai Tea afterwards. LOL

* I schedule video chats when "in person" isn't possible.

* How about leaving handwritten notes of appreciation on someone's desk or in their coat pocket to be found at some unexpected time? A sentence or two is enough. We have lost this basic kindness to show others they are appreciated.

Also, recognize that things may have changed for you. You have gone through a 5-week journey *so far* of improving your health. Where are some *new opportunities to increase your social engagement*?

Maybe things have been changing in your body and mind, and now maybe there are experiences that are available to you that weren't before. For example:

* Maybe you are now able to walk longer (endurance) and can join that forest walk with your friends.

* Maybe you are now more comfortable in your body and therefore more able to connect with other people and go to that beach picnic.

* Maybe you can now build social connections through activities you couldn't try before, like Tai Chi classes.

* Maybe you are now motivated to join a new cooking class to advance your repertoire of healthy meals.

* Maybe you now have increased self-confidence and energy to do the inviting instead of waiting to be invited.

* Maybe you have other hobbies and interests you can pursue now: get more involved in political activism, take an art class, teach a skill you possess at your local community centre, or volunteer. All these things will connect you with an expanding tribe.

Are you ready to EXPAND YOUR TRIBE? New Friendships 101:

New friendships are exciting and stimulating as you are exposed to new perspectives, new opportunities for growth and adventure. The basis for creating new friendships rests on a few fundamental questions:

* Do I trust this person?
* Do I respect this person?
* Do we share common values?

There need to be beneficial qualities:

* Multiple opportunities to connect in different environments (social events, rituals, celebrations)
* A practice of vulnerability (a foundation of strong relationships)
* A positive optimism since emotions are contagious
* A competition for kindness

YOUR TURN: Homework Time

Look at the areas of Deep Connections skills; where is your main opportunity (eliminate or reduce the impact of harmful relationships; strengthen your valuable relationships; build new connections)? Choose

ONE thing you will do this week to strengthen your Deep Connections toolbox. If you have a level one practice already, try a level two or three.

Action steps/habit building

Level One: *Evaluate and clear space* (if needed)

* List your top 3+ people you can count on in life for fun and support (sometimes it's nice to write down what you appreciate about the person and the relationship to remind yourself of gratitude).

* Any tough decisions? Do you need to let go of or scale down a relationship? How will you do that? Outline the first baby step you can take.

Level Two: *Enhance current relationships*

* Which of your relationships need enhancements?

* Choose one step this week to increase your social connections.

* Make a plan in your schedule to connect with these people at least every week.

* Choose your engagement activities and write them in your weekly calendar.

* Make this part of your daily schedule this week.

Level Three: *Make new connections*

* Which new opportunities are you open to in order to expand your tribe?

* Join new groups, start new clubs.

WHAT IS NEXT?

You got it: All this sounds simple, but it takes practice. Strengthening this area rewards us the most in our health and our happiness. Address the area first that you feel will yield you the best results. Start with baby steps. Remember, changing too much too quickly is NOT sustainable. You can always add more when you are able to maintain and ready to scale up in this category. When you adopt level one practices, move on to level two and three as you are ready.

Ok, now you have your tribe... Let's go just a little deeper. Next week... What's **the point** of *all* this...?

CHAPTER 9

WHAT'S YOUR POINT?

Week 7: **Sense of Purpose**

*"We are here to fulfill our unique purpose, mission, career, role...
to discover your story, stay true to it and act from it."*
Vishen Lakhiani

Another of the pillars of health and longevity, as the *National Institute of Aging* states, is having a strong sense of purpose in our lives. The things that bring meaning to your days and your life overall. Your POINT for doing things. I lost my purpose for a bit there, and I felt quite lost. "What am I doing? What's the point of doing it?" was my prevalent thought. But it can be easier than you think to get back on track.

Once I rediscovered my purpose, all the synchronicities started showing up. Coincidences. Things my brain was now focused on looking for that would help me along my path. The right people started showing up for me at the right time. People who could help me advance my purpose. I'd ask myself a question about where to go for XYZ, and suddenly a new resource was there. Things began falling into place. Once we are aligned with our purpose, the universe helps guide us along the path. It becomes easy.

What's your purpose? Your point for doing things? For example, why are you here? Still reading...still creating habits? Still wanting more?

It's an interesting question. WHY? You started reading this book for a reason... WHAT was that reason? What were you wanting? What was the **purpose** behind your actions? Something motivated you to make a change, to take action. That's what a sense of purpose does. It motivates. It is your WHY. Your compass.

If you know your purpose in life, YAY YOU! When your motivation wanes, remind yourself often of your WHYs, your reason for doing things. Some of these next ideas may help you do that on an even deeper level. If you aren't sure at this point what your purpose is and how to find it, you can start here.

HOW DO WE DO THIS?

1.   Define Your WHYS
2.   Map Your Values
3.   Choose Your Action

1.   DEFINE YOUR WHYS

Let's start by thinking: WHY do you do things? Why do any of us do anything? Psychology tells us it is usually either to gain a reward or to avoid a negative consequence.

For example, in terms of your health journey, you likely either wanted to experience something positive (a kayak trip down the river) or avoid a negative outcome (developing diabetes). Our reasons shape our values, which largely shape our decisions about things. What is important to you? What matters?

For me, having both my parents die quite young from preventable diseases, it matters to me to be here for my son and to be healthy for as long as possible.

There are reasons you chose to work on your own health. What result were you wanting? Were you wanting to inspire your family to make healthier choices by changing some of your own practices? Were you wanting to be able to crawl around on the floor with your grandkids? Maybe you wanted to start your own business and needed energy and clarity of mind to do so.

Consider your sense of purpose around your health journey. Explore and record your thoughts here. Ask yourself why. This is fuel for your motivation. Remember the **FOGG Method: MAP** (motivation, ability, prompt). We always start with MOTIVATION! Make it strong inside your mind. In the next chapter, we will look at how to make these changes sustainable and integrate them with your identity while the rest of *life* happens around you.

But let's think for a minute above and beyond your health. Our health is our car, our vehicle that carries us through life's experiences. What experiences are *you* wanting in life? It's sort of like that age-old question: *Why are we here?*

This is a question we have pondered through the ages. But more specifically, why are **YOU** here? What purpose is there in your life? It might seem like a confrontational question, I suppose. I don't mean it that way. It's just that we all chose this human experience... What was it we wanted to learn while we were here? What is it we want to share and pass on before we leave?

Your sense of purpose, finding meaning in your life, is related to **Maslow's Hierarchy fourth and fifth tier**: (self-esteem and self-actualization) *feeling valued and knowing your life has meaning*. We are more motivated for just about anything in life if we have a beneficial purpose in mind.

Remember that set of questions from the *National Institute of Aging*? The ones that indicate how long and how well you may live? **"Do you have a sense of purpose that gives meaning to your life?"**

At certain times in your life, your life's purpose may have been different. I, for example, spent the past 3 decades as a public school teacher working in the inner city with some of our most vulnerable learners. This was my purpose, which arose from my values, which were created from my experience. My experience as a child of "needing" some adult as a role model created my values: I wanted kids to have a better experience than I had. My purpose was to make that happen by working skillfully and compassionately with vulnerable youth. My WHY motivated me to do that and to do it very well. I turned my "values" into a career.

Now, as my career role is changing, I understand it is because a new value has taken hold of me. My purpose now is in sharing what I've learned and supporting as many people as I can (kids, adults, everyone) to make a health revolution and live our happiest and healthiest lives. Kids are still important to me. I hope, if all of us adults can learn to be healthier role models, their future will be positively impacted. They are watching, and they do copy... even if they deny it.

We can deepen or expand our WHYs by defining our values. This helps to reinforce *our motivation for action.* What is it you want and why?

Maybe your purpose is in being there for your children and grandchildren as fully capable as possible. Maybe it's developing your own business that serves the world. Maybe it's to teach others the skills you have learned from a lifetime of experience in a particular area.

2.   MAP YOUR VALUES

Your values shape the decisions you make in your life.

> *"Until you make the unconscious conscious,*
> *it will direct your life and you will call it fate."*
> Carl Jung

The more aware you are of your values, the easier it will be for you to make decisions aligned with that purpose. So, what are your values? What fulfills you? How do you want to grow? What can you uniquely offer the world?

When you start to make time for inner stillness and listen to your authentic inner voice, you will begin to understand what your soul is here to do in this world at this time. Heavy stuff? Sure! But...seriously, it is the WHY of EVERYTHING!!! Why do anything at all otherwise? Our lives are MEANT to have meaning. And each one of us has unique gifts necessary in the world; we are all pieces of the puzzle, creating a masterpiece by design.

Do you know your values? Sometimes you get a trigger...a place, a person, a concept you are drawn to for no apparent reason. These can be clues. Things or experiences that compel you.

> *"Your values were deliberately placed within your soul. They are the seeds of*
> *what the universe is seeking to create through you.*
> *Listen carefully to what is emerging."*
> Vishen Lakhiani

I believe, as *Vishen Lakhani* explains in his book **The Buddha and the Badass**, that we each have "soulprint", unique markers for our soul based on the experiences our soul seeks to have in this lifetime. He goes on to say that when you listen to your authentic voice:

> *"...you will understand what your soul is actually driven to do in this world. And this is the reason you were truly born....(pg28)*
> *"Your values were deliberately placed with your soul. They are the seeds of what the Universe is seeking to create through you. Listen carefully to what's emerging." (pg41)*

Often, these values get formed during early childhood and adolescent learning periods. Traumatic events often shape our lives; they drive us to choose or choose not certain behaviours. Usually, it stems from something painful; this is where we are motivated to change the most. For example, I vowed as a teacher to leave my school by 3:30 so I could be available to my own child after that...because I was stranded til past midnight with my mother at school or pawned off on other families to care for me for days because she was too busy working.

Vishen's technique on how to map your values:

* *Explore your past:* Values often come from painful things because that is when we make powerful decisions about how we will behave in the future. But values could also come from great highs in our lives as well.

* What was the story? What happened? How did you feel?

* GO through age 5-25. Write the values that came from these moments.

* What is the most painful moment you experienced as a child? What was your greatest high?

    OR

* Chart your highs and lows of childhood? Remember some of the most painful parts.

* What was the important part? List what matters to you in life that arises from those memories.

* Find the common themes from your list. Cluster the list into main categories.

* Name these categories...these are your values.

This can be tough work. It can bring up a lot of feelings. I now have many strategies to deal with past shadows. But if you need additional support, please consult your medical professionals.

"You can't connect the dots looking forward; you can only connect them looking backwards. So, you have to trust that the dots will somehow connect in your future. You have to trust in something – you gut, destiny, life, karma, whatever. This approach has never let me down and it has made all the difference in my life."
Steve Jobs 2005

3.   **CHOOSE YOUR ACTION**: What will your contribution be?

Now, after mapping your values, what does it reflect to you? What shows up that fulfills you and makes you want to grow? What can you uniquely offer the world?

Think of all your life experiences. In the end, what is the meaning of all that? What have you experienced? What have you learned? What have you shared? We are meant to share our knowledge. Who would have ever been touched by or benefited by it all if you kept things only onto yourself? What's the point of learning if you can't share it with others? It is how our species survived.

"It's what teach from what you learn. It's what you provide from what you get. It's what you facilitate from what you experience... it's what gives meaning to the convergence part. There is No meaning for you to learn things if you are not teaching. There is no meaning in learning if you are not teaching. There is no meaning in experiencing if you are not facilitating. No meaning for you to get if you are not providing. And this is your time now to honour all the converging experiences into transcending yourself and reaching out to others."
Ronan Diego de Oliveira

Are we here just to have fun and exploit the nature and beauty in the world? I don't think so...

We learn...and we share. That's how our species survived thus far. Are we meeting those needs now? How can you contribute, share your experience and knowledge to help other living things? We are here to serve...ourselves and others: To contribute to humanity in a positive way; to leave a place better than we found it; to look after living things and the gift of nature; and to learn and to share our knowledge with others.

Where do you fit in this story? What are you offering the world?

Now, after mapping out your values and what sparks excitement for further growth and looking more into what you have experienced and learned, it's time to decide: *What are you in the unique position of sharing with others to benefit their life?* How can you contribute to a happy, healthy, positive world? Because isn't that really why we are here? To learn and grow and contribute to a better world? I think so! Your job is to figure out how you fit in.

YOUR TURN: Homework Time

Look at the 3 areas of Sense of Purpose skills; where is your main opportunity (Define your WHYs, map your values, choose your actions and make a contribution)? Choose ONE thing you will do this week to strengthen your inner stillness toolbox. If you have a level one practice already, try a level two or three.

Action steps/habit building

Level One: *Define your WHYs*

* Record why you started this health journey. Keep this list handy and remind yourself of it often.

*List any other reasons WHY you do things that you are aware of.

Level Two: *Map your values*

* Explore times in your early life. What difficult events were there? What beliefs did you create around that? What values do you see emerging from this list? What matters to you?

Level Three: *Choose your actions*

* Explore your learning in life and think about how your knowledge could benefit someone else.

* How can you make a contribution?

* What action can you take around this area?

* Decide one action you will take this week that is aligned with your sense of purpose in life.

WHAT'S NEXT?

You can probably recite this with me by now... All this sounds simple, but it takes practice. Address the area first that you feel will yield you the best results. Start with baby steps. Remember, changing too much too quickly is NOT sustainable. You can always add more when you are able to maintain and ready to scale up in this category. When you adopt level one practices, move on to level two and three as you are ready.

And now...with a 7-week journey under your belt, you may be wondering: *What's next?*

And without further adieu, I will see you next week for our last **"What's Next?"**

CHAPTER 10

LATHER. RINCE. REPEAT.

Week 8 and Beyond: **What's Next?**

At this point in the journey, after 7 weeks, we have implemented a lot of new habits and practices to achieve a state of baseline health and fitness. You may now be experiencing one of two things:

1. You've implemented a lot and are starting to feel the difference.
2. You're overwhelmed by the amount of tools.

Both are totally normal. Wherever you are right now is FANTASTIC! This process can go on indefinitely by adding new habits and having a progressive focus on current habits. This is a JOURNEY, not a destination.

Remember, you **don't** have to be perfect at everything in order to move forward. Don't get yourself stuck here by trying to nail everything perfectly. Let's work on some sustainability practices to ensure lasting change. Let's go back to WHY.

Here we are *again* with WHY! Why are you here? Still reading...still creating habits? Still wanting more?

It's an interesting and invaluable question. WHY? You started for a reason... WHAT was that reason? What were you wanting? Something **sustainable**, I would imagine. And where we need to go now is a little deeper. How do we make things we have gained *sustainable*? We begin by again looking at our reasons to care.

What is the *story* you told yourself in the beginning...? What *vision* did you have for yourself? Why did you care about that?

"I wanted to feel _____".

"I wanted to be able to _____".

At this stage, we want to activate those visions again and make them part of our identity. We want *sustainability. I.E., How do we create lasting change?* First, we start with creating a *Story Vision.*

STORY VISION

Creating a Story Vision is much more compelling than just a statement. We are hardwired to understand stories. Our story vision is what helps us keep moving forward in the journey to maintain and improve our health. It is our reason to care, our motivation for action.

Think about your perfect day...moment to moment. What really matters to you? What do you want to feel? What do you want to be able to do? What do you want to achieve? What do you want to look and be like? What *experiences* do you want to have? Brainstorm some words and concepts here.

From these moments, we create our goals. But our vision of a compelling and exciting future is the motivational force that drives our actions. This story should be:

* **Grounded**, doable, and possible. You can't grow wings and fly.

* Yet it should also be a bit **audacious**, unreasonable, to go beyond the average, *to be exciting.*

* It should be **genuine,** something you truly want, not what others want for you.

* It should be **transcendental**; to go beyond yourself to touch others' lives.

* It should be **tangible** and easily understood, like in story form.

Once we have spent time creating our story visions, goals, and actions, how do we make sure that the vision stays alive for us while the rest of our life happens?

INTEGRATING OUR STORY VISION WITH OUR IDENTITY FOR LASTING CHANGE

There is a moment before having a meal that is very powerful. Many cultures have a mindful practice at this time of day. You are about to nurture your body with life force. It is a recognition that we are about to absorb energy in order to manifest things we want to experience in our lives. Take a moment here to remember what it is that you are trying to manifest.

Use that moment before a meal to remind yourself of one of the moments in your story vision. The more you recall your stories, the more they become integrated into your identity. Your brain doesn't know the difference between rehearsal and reality...so "practice" your story. The more we do this, the more effortless the actions towards it become because they start to blend into our self-identity. I call this my MVP time **(Mealtime Visualization Practice).**

SAFETY NETS

Use **Safety Nets** when you feel resistance. Define the minimum version of a habit that you still consider a success.

For example, when it rains in the morning, I occasionally have resistance to doing my morning walk habit. The thought of 30 minutes and getting soaked becomes daunting. I don't "feel like" doing it. But I create a safety net (I will just walk around the block). Do the smallest version of the habit. So, if your morning routine takes an hour and a half, maybe your safety net is 15 minutes. Maybe instead of a 30-minute walk, you will walk to the end of the street and come back. Maybe you do one rep of each exercise in your training session instead of 25.

By doing the minimum version of the habit, you are still strengthening the habit behaviour, which creates shifts in your self-identity. It becomes a thought in your mind: "This is what I do."

When you do at least a small version of the habit that you are building, you create the "real estate" for the habit to happen. The time is allocated. However, sometimes when I decide to do the safety net version, once I have started and created the "space" for the routine... I just keep going. It's like how they used to say, "Just put your workout gear in the bag and drive to the gym. You don't have to work out." Then, inevitably, once you're there, you go inside and do the workout anyways. Taking *some* action creates motivation for further action. But do at least the bare minimum. **A *habit missed once is an accident; a habit missed twice is the start of a new habit.***

Creating A Safety Net Routine:

* Define the **Safety Net** = the minimum version of the habit that you consider a success.

* Remember *Zero Resistance Habits*... what is the easiest version or step of the habit that you can perform? *It is much **harder to restart** a habit you gave up on entirely **than to expand** on a habit you are doing. Keep doing the minimum version, if nothing else.*

* Look at your whole daily routine; what are the habits you are implementing?

* Create the safety net for all the habits you are trying to implement. Make it crazy small. It doesn't have to give you a long-term health benefit; it just needs to happen. Nurturing this habit is what will bring long-term health benefits.

HABIT	Minimum Version / Safety Net

GET BACK UP Prompt

There will always be moments of "falling off the wagon", moments of "failures". It is normal, it is expected...and it is amazing when it happens. Why? Well, because It gives us the opportunity to get back up. The important thing is to keep getting back up and do it quickly.

114

Remember, *one missed day is an accident. Two missed days is the start of a new habit.*

In martial arts combat training, there is an element where you lay down and practice getting back up quickly. If you assume that you will never get knocked down in combat and you only practice your kicks and punches, you will have trouble getting back up quickly when it inevitably happens. If you don't practice getting back up, you have no skill to do it when you need to.

Life happens…. Assume things will happen and prepare yourself to deal with them without throwing yourself off course. "Failures" are opportunities to get back up quickly. When I falter, I clap my hands twice and say, "Wake up" or "Back in the game" (it reframes my focus).

Creating A "Get Back UP" prompt
("Failures" are your opportunity to get back up quickly)

* Identify **WHERE** you fell. Create awareness for future prevention.

* Identify **HOW** you get back up (this creates a reset in your mind vs just throwing in the towel completely). Make it a small little habit… like our celebration habit. A gesture, a phrase.

So…PHEW!

We're coming to the end of a 7-week journey. I am so grateful to have had you join me on this path, and I hope you feel inspired to continue growing, learning, and improving. It isn't complicated, but it isn't always easy either. You are already a superhero for battling all the forces against you!

So far, we have adopted new habits that establish a baseline of health and fitness and will continue to improve our level of health and fitness *even if we do nothing more*. Celebrate yourself and all that you have achieved this far!!

Let's reflect and evaluate here by asking ourselves:

115

1. What is your attitude towards your body now?

I now see my body as a partner. I give it what it needs, protect it from harm, and nurture its innate gifts. I appreciate its resiliency and how it reacts well to change. I have stopped pushing its limits and value it more. *What about you?*

2. What are you grateful for?

I am grateful for creating time to focus on myself, for my guides and mentors along the learning journey, for visible results that lead people to ask for guidance, and for finding a second life calling through this journey. *How about you?*

3. How is this journey you're on making you closer to other people going forward?

Maybe you can squat down to play with your grandchild now. Maybe you feel lighter and freer and able to start practicing a sport. Maybe you're developing a habit of cooking and can prepare meals for others and teach others. Maybe you're more comfortable in social environments (to control food, restaurant plans, go to the beach, or travel). Make a list of all the gifts you have given yourself in the past 7 weeks that now make interactions and transcendence of your own journey into connection with other people easier, better, and more available.

4. What battles did you win, or what challenges did you overcome?

In these 7 weeks, there were things that you achieved, things that you learned. There were battles that you won (even if they weren't the ones you were intending to win in the beginning). Maybe you think, "I still haven't achieved XYZ goal..." Yes, perhaps, but take time to identify and appreciate what you HAVE done. This might lead you to see who you can support and who you can help with what you've learned. Maybe it's your kids, your grandkids, our future generations.

Whatever battles you win, there are others around you who are starting their battle right now, and you can help them. *What were your wins?*

5. What was your toughest episode?

Mine came about in week 12 of an intense 16-week program. I was experiencing overwhelm, lost momentum, and was worried that what I had worked so hard to build would fall apart. But with the *Safety Net and Get Back Up* tools, I kept on moving forward. *What was toughest for you?*

6. The important part: What was the lesson in it?

For me, I learned things aren't black and white. You don't fail or succeed. You move forward with kindness and baby steps. Life happens. Don't quit. Adapt and overcome. *What was your lesson?*

7. What are the battles that are still to be won?

Maybe you didn't achieve one of the goals you had in the beginning. Or maybe new battles arose as you went through each stage. Maybe there are other things you want to try or other things you want to learn. These will be your next journeys. For me, I am still refining my *Wind Down routine. What are you still working on?*

8. What tools/practices made a difference for you?

For me, the morning routine, strength training, tracking for progression, intermittent fasting and elimination diet, tracking biomarkers for feedback and motivation, the Safety Net and Get Back Up strategies made the biggest impact. Also, for me, giving up sugar made a HUGE difference, as did giving up dairy, grains, and caffeine. *What has made a difference for you so far?*

9. How will you apply what you've learned?

I decided to become certified to teach what I've learned to anyone who's interested. I want to help expand the health revolution: a healthier planet with healthier, happier people. *What will you do?*

TIME TO *DECIDE* WHAT'S NEXT.

You have some choices to make:

1. Do you want to move to a "**Maintenance Mode**", gently following the 7 habits with lots of flexibility?

2. Are you ready to keep working on your "Baseline health and fitness", starting a **new 7 week cycle**, and adopting more habits for continual scaling up?

3. Are you wanting to try to challenge yourself for accelerated transformation by starting a "**Rapid Acceleration Mode**"?

MAINTENANCE MODE

Continuing on with what you have built this far is awesome! You are on the right track for helping your body thrive, giving your body what it needs, protecting it from harm, and nurturing its innate gifts. This will go a long way to increasing your immune system and all the processes your body needs to perform in order for it to heal itself and stay at peak levels of health.

A *maintenance mode* is more about giving the body permission to express what it wants to become. It is a low-structured plan and is about listening to what your body wants and needs. It is a great phase for sustainability.

If you do nothing else but continue with the habits you have adopted thus far, you are winning!

However, when you are ready and decide it's time to scale up for continuous improvements, all you need to do is go back to the 7 habits and choose an action on the next level.

START A NEW 7 WEEK CYCLE

Each of the 7 habits we have covered has some suggestions for action steps at different levels of the game. Level One (beginning steps),

Two (intermediate steps), and Three (more advanced actions). Go back and find a next-level action you can adopt. Listen to your body. What actions does it want you to take next?

If you aren't sure where to start, look at all the habits and evaluate your current state:

* Are you FAR from your goal (1),
* MEDIUM range from your goal (2), or
* CLOSE to your goal (3) ?

Next, look at your level of action in that area:

* Are you taking HIGH action (1,)
* MEDIUM action (2), or
* LOW action (3) ?

Choose a habit to work on from a *medium-range state and low action*. It's too big a jump to work on a far-range habit with low action. Baby steps are what create sustainability!

It might look like this:

Habits	Current State	Current Action
Sound Sleep	Med	low
Nutrient Richness	Close	med
Frequent Movement	Med	low
Sync with Nature	Close	high
Inner Stillness	Far	high
Deep Connections	Close	low
Sense of Purpose	Med	high

By this assessment, you'd work on *Sound Sleep* or *Frequent Movement.*

RAPID ACCELERATION MODE

If you are ready and looking for an accelerated transformation, there is so much to explore that it cannot be covered within the scope

119

of this book. It includes taking biomarkers, tracking, progressive acceleration training routines, strategic nutrition, and more. It is a sprint. It is not sustainable long term but is done with a specific goal and timeframe in mind.

I am including a list of some of the concepts and skills that I have learned and employed to accelerate my own transformation. This type of adventure is best done with support to manage obstacles that come up, to help guide and monitor progress, to help guide adjustments, and to encourage. Acceleration modes are geared to be *temporary accelerated actions targeted for specific results*. It's intense. But it raises the bar for what's possible for you. By doing things that are hard, we make the hard easier.

And, if you are wanting even more...

I've done a lot of research, learned a lot of strategies, and gained a lot of credentials. I have created support programs designed to help people at all stages of the journey, from just starting to revamp their health, to those working on advanced fitness. I offer everything from a 7-day program to 6-month advanced-level training courses. All are accessible in a small group setting or as individual one on one programs. If you'd like any more support with your journey, I'd love to see you in one of our group programs or in an individualized session.

As they say: *"If you want to go fast, go alone. If you want to go far, go together."*

YOUR TURN: Last Homework Time

Level One:

* Write your story vision:
> Write out your Perfect Day. Write all the moments.

Write out your top 5 reasons to care about your Story vision. (E.g., I truly care about my story vision because my sporting choices will be more abundant when I have more mobility, I will be here longer for my son, I will feel pride at my choices and accomplishments, I will connect more with others because I am abundantly energetic, and I will have energy for whatever I want to do in life.)

Now pick a milestone on the journey. A kayak trip? A mini marathon? A travel adventure? A business goal? Make it a specific outcome. Make it challenging. What is the moment you want to **experience**? This moment is powered by your reason to care. What is possible because of your actions?

Find 4 more moments along your journey. Is it buying a new bike? Is it kayaking down a river? Is it playing with your grandkids on a family vacation? Is it writing a blog post to inspire others?

From there, you find your goals and can effectively choose your actions.

1. What do you want to experience? (I want to have a healthy body to hike with my kids)
2. What is the root cause of that desire? (I want to be independent and share adventures)
3. What is at stake if you don't achieve that? (I will be dependent on others and die early)
4. What do you NOT want? (to starve myself, smoke, drink often, and die early of a stroke like my dad, nor to eat junk, never move my body, and die of cancer early like my mother)

* Create your **Safety Net Routine** for each of your new habits

* Design your **Get Back Up** Strategy
Level Two:

* MVP - Meal Time Visualization Practice
a. Take 6 deep **breathes** to activate the parasympathetic nervous system
b. Visualize the actions happening and experience the **feelings** you will have at that moment when you achieve it
c. Express **gratitude** for being in this place
d. **Visualize** the action steps it will take to get there
e. Create a little **mantra/prayer** (e.g., let it be so, amen, etc.)

* **Habits**: remind yourself of what you're trying to accomplish by visualizing often and over time. The more you visualise it, the more it becomes part of your self-identity.

Level Three:

* Reflect on your journey.

* Decide what's next for you: a maintenance mode, a new 7-week cycle, or an acceleration mode.

If it's a **maintenance mode**: keep on truckin' and enjoy all the benefits you feel from what you have achieved by implementing new habits and routines to promote a healthy lifestyle and the best version of yourself that you can be. YAY, You!!! Enjoy the experience. It's a journey...not a destination.

I encourage you to be your own expert. This is a self-driven journey of learning. Keep researching new areas; find more movement activities, new recipes, new nature locations to visit, and new ways to connect with others. Life is learning. Maintenance mode is all about what is sustainable and what is enjoyable.

If you're ready, start a **New 7-week cycle**. Go back and observe. What level of action steps did you take this go around in each of the 7 habits? If you did a Level One action step for a Frequent Movement habit, try a level two action step this time around. Choose a next-level action step for each of the 7 habits as you move through the 7-week cycle. Remember to track where you start and throughout the process. Monitoring progress and noting improvements is the motivation fuel here.

If you decide you are ready for an accelerated transformation, a **Rapid Acceleration Mode**, there are many components for further study:

- More on elimination diets
- Intermittent fasting
- Functional fitness
- Compound exercises
- Mechanical tension, muscular fatigue, progression overload

- Exercise/"working out" VS Training (i.e., a structured program designed for targeted results for a specific goal)
- Optimizing fitness training
- Women's issue focus on training (training during menstrual cycles, pre or post-menopause etc.)
- Hormonal balances
- The Hormonal Hierarchy
- Sleep optimization
- Calorie Intake and the CICO Model vs. The Insulin Model
- Energy balance overview
- Macronutrient design
- Micronutrient design
- Master meal design
- Environmental design
- Eliminating more endocrine disruptors
- Building morning and evening routines

A brief note on generalized needs during **menopause** (Always seek medical advice or specialized support where needed):

* There is decreased estrogen production which reduces the BMR over time, leading to weight gain. Try eating foods with decreased calorie density, increase your protein intake, or try low carb – high-fat diet design.

* There is decreased progesterone production; therefore, increased chronic stress can happen, leading to irritability and mood swings. Try to outsource responsibilities where possible, delegate, employ your support networks, take magnesium, and use paced breathing.

* There is a higher risk of osteoporosis from lack of estrogen production. Try more strength training.

WHAT'S NEXT?

Remember this from the beginning?

"The number one thing people do wrong is to try to make too many changes too quickly. We rush the first steps. There is a sense of urgency that we need to make the changes yesterday because we've let things go to the point that we are desperate. We can't keep up with all the rapid changes, so we give up on changing our lifestyles. This is a sign of unconscious transformation. We need to decrease the sense of urgency and realise this is a continuous journey. Keep doing 1% improvements."

Scale up or down, you can't change everything all at once. Choose one thing to start with, or you'll burn out. Anticipate that life WILL get in the way sometimes. Your "best" might differ from day to day. When things get busy, instead of completely skipping your habit, continue to leave space for it to happen, even at a minimal level. By maintaining the space for your habit, you continue to reinforce consistency.

Remember, it's not about being perfect, checking off all the boxes each day, and reaching a final destination. Your best is different from day to day. Life happens. Use your **Safety Nets** and your **Get Back Up routine.** You don't need to be perfect to move on to the next steps (don't get bogged down with all the minutia and details). It is a journey of a lifetime... Enjoy it!

Keep growing, keep improving! Be healthy, be happy!
Lather. Rince. Repeat.

For more information on courses or services offered please visit:

https://www.workwithtam.ca/

Know what you want next? Use the code **"READ7"** for a **discount on all programs and services**

Want to give up sugar? 7 day program info:
https://www.workwithtam.ca/sugar-shakedown

Want to be trained in the Silva Ultramind Method for healing?
https://www.workwithtam.ca/silva

Want a complete mind/body reset? 8 weeks to a new you!
https://www.workwithtam.ca/reset-recharge

Want more info about the 6 Phase Meditation or to discuss a personalized journey? Book a free clarity call and I can answer all your questions:
https://www.workwithtam.ca/services or email me at Tam@workwithtam.ca

See you soon ☺

Made in the USA
Columbia, SC
29 November 2023

b12c8f86-0018-4211-8dd4-1bc4f82a95f7R01